P9-BIO-366

". . . professionals, patients, partners, parents-to-be, or any concerned citizen can benefit from this authoritative book."

> *Dr. Gordon Jessamine,*
> *Chairman, Sexually Transmitted Diseases Division,*
> *Canadian Public Health Association*

"For those who only wish to purchase one [book], I would suggest that patients with genital herpes read *The Truth About Herpes.*"

> *excerpt from* Sexually Transmitted Diseases,
> *journal of the American Venereal Disease Association*

"In tackling popular myths and misconceptions about herpes simplex virus, Dr. Sacks' talent for metaphor and wit sets the facts straight in a manner that not only appeals to the general reader, but leaves a lasting impression and a scientifically correct one at that. His writing balances technical accuracy, humor, insights from clinical experience with patients, and self-confessed 'professional bias'. In a clearly personal, yet scientifically competent tone, he has put together a comprehensive book on herpes written in unusually appealing language."

> *excerpt from* The Helper,
> *a publication of the Herpes Resource Center*
> *(For the past decade, the Herpes Resource Center has*
> *been North America's primary source of reliable*
> *information about herpes, and has served as the*
> *international resource agency for herpes self-help chapters*
> *in 100 cities.)*

THE TRUTH ABOUT HERPES

Third Edition

by

Stephen L. Sacks, M.D.

Founder and Director
University of British Columbia
Herpes Clinic

Gordon Soules Book Publishers Ltd.
West Vancouver, Canada
Seattle, U.S.A.

Copyright © 1988 by Stephen L. Sacks
Fifth printing of third edition January, 1991

All rights reserved. No part of this book may be
reproduced in any form by any means without the
written permission of the publisher, except by a reviewer,
who may quote passages in a review.

Canadian Cataloguing in Publication Data

Sacks, Stephen L., 1948—
    The truth about herpes

    Bibliography: p.
    Includes index.
    ISBN 0-919574-58-0

    1. Herpes simplex.   I. Title.
    RC203.H45S33   1987   616.95'18   C88-091050-X

Published in Canada by
Gordon Soules Book Publishers Ltd.
1352-B Marine Drive
West Vancouver, B.C.
Canada   V7T 1B5

Published in the U.S.A. by
Gordon Soules Book Publishers Ltd.
620 - 1916 Pike Place
Seattle, WA 98101

Cover illustration by Eroca Brawne
Typesetting by Joy Woodsworth and The Typeworks
Printed and bound in Canada by Hignell Printing Limited

For Anne and Leon
For Marika
For Adrian and Rebecca
For Krystyna

CONTENTS

ACKNOWLEDGMENTS

I would like to express thanks to my coworkers at the Herpes Clinic and the Infectious Diseases Laboratory at the University of British Columbia, past and present, who have made this book possible. They have provided the counseling, administered the research, worked with the cell cultures and the new drugs, and coped with the personal crises and the funding fluctuations. Without them, there would be no experience to share with you. They are Dr. H. Grant Stiver, P. Lynn Buhler, Rebecca Fox, Paul Levendusky, Nancy Ruedy, Terri Varner, Megan O'Connor, Pam Brewis, Kim Davies, Marion Barker, Marika Sacks, Maureen Barfoot, Laurel Lemchuk-Favel, Chong Ze-Teh, Mike Ashe, Shaun Culham, Paula Galloway, Jim Wanklin, Susan Rayner, Joyce Diggins, and Elda Wilson.

Marguerite Drummond and Bruce Stewart did the line illustrations. K. Wong and Dr. D. McLean supplied the electron micrograph. John Graves and the Herpes Resource Center were absolutely essential in the evolution and success of this book. Tom Bell and Lou Kozak gave this book its freedom. Dr. Michael Rosenberg of the American Social Health Association, Guy Lallemand of the Ortho Pharmaceutical (Canada), Ltd., and Anne-Louise Gibbins assisted me with research in preparing the new chapter on condoms. Astra Pharmaceuticals and the Canadian Public Health Association helped to get the first edition off the ground. Marika Sacks served as editor, added the chapter quotations, advised on content, translated many of my thoughts into coherent English, balanced the ledgers, and believed in me. I thank you all.

Most of all, I thank my patients, who have given their blood,

Acknowledgments

their pictures, and their cultures for my teaching and research. They have given me the reasons to teach about herpes and to seek new methods for treatment. They have shared with me their secrets, their pains, their joys, and their thanks.

INTRODUCTION

If I have herpes does that make me a sexual leper? Is herpes a sign of the Apocalypse? Is it the wrath of God? A modern-day plague? Will I be able to have children if I get it? Will it give me cancer? Is it incurable? Should I become celibate? Should I see a divorce lawyer? Will I go blind? Is this an incurable social disease that deforms babies and causes cancer? These concerns, and many more, are real ones for the thousands of people whose lives are touched by herpes. The questions are numerous, and they keep coming. Answers are essential.

At the University of British Columbia Herpes Clinic we have seen thousands of people with genital herpes infections. We have listened carefully to thousands of questions and done our best to answer them with facts. A glance at the table of contents will give you an idea of what people are asking. Many questions come up again and again. The answers are based on current medical knowledge as well as day-by-day clinical experience.

There is no question that herpes is a growing problem. The number of people affected is increasing at an alarming rate. Unfortunately, misinformation has increased along with the growth rate. We do not know just how many people are affected with herpes, but guesses of 500,000 to 1,000,000 *new* cases in North America per year have been made. These figures are generally based on how many people with herpes go to clinics that treat sexually transmitted diseases. However, all people with herpes do not necessarily go to such clinics. Family doctors as well as specialists in dermatology, urology, gynecology, or infectious diseases are diagnosing and treating herpes. Furthermore, because herpes is not always diagnosed with a standard lab test and because it is not a "notifiable" disease like syphilis or tuberculosis, there are no dependable statistics. During the last decade the number of people seeking medical attention for this problem has increased more than tenfold.

Along with the rise in incidence of genital herpes, there has been a parallel upswing in media attention. Some have suggested that the problem has grown more in print than on people's skin. While there is an element of truth in this feeling, herpes remains all too real to the person who has it. It is a serious concern to anyone who is or who plans to be sexually active in his or her life, whether those plans include one lifetime partner or a hundred. Coping with and living a normal life *around* herpes is a challenge that can be met. To meet this challenge, however, you must arm yourself with the truth. Unfortunately, the dissemination of useful information has not always been the goal in the recent media obsession with herpes. For television and newspapers, herpes has become a major news event—from public affairs shows to the eleven o'clock news, from exposé glossies to weekly news magazines. Such unrelenting public exposure to the problem actually changed the disease itself. One might be left with the impression that herpes is no longer a problem, since the media no longer address it. *Time* magazine stayed only long enough to label herpes the "Scarlet Letter." The positive aspects of the media hype are gone, i.e., the educational component and the pressure for research funding. Yet because of the attention focused on genital herpes in the early 1980s, it is no longer just a sexually transmitted infection that requires understanding—it has become a stigma which requires destigmatizing.

Television programs, magazines, and even books wholly devoted to herpes have only rarely dealt with the subject with care. From the personal anecdotes told at cocktail parties to the summaries in seventy words printed next to an ad for perfume, the issues surrounding this common infection have all too often been dealt with in a haphazard fashion. Even the medical profession has had a tough job of it. The time required to inform the patient fully about the problem, explain the details, and answer the questions is not always available in the doctor's office.

Several good organizations have been formed to help provide reliable information about herpes, but unless you're aware that they exist, they can't be of any help. Most of what's in print about herpes avoids the difficult questions, talking about the subject only in a superficial way. This book is different. It will take you step-by-step through the plain facts. Your fears surrounding herpes will be honestly met—nothing, pleasant or unpleasant, is glossed over. Yet the truth has a way of placing fears into perspective. If you are reading this book to learn whether you have herpes, read on. It is important that you do find out, and this book will tell you how to do just that. If you are reading it to find a method for prevention, read on. You may not find a simple answer to the question, but you will know enough to approach prevention intelligently. If you are reading this book to find out about treatment, read on. A new drug makes it possible for the first time to control this infection, but the treatment is not for everybody. If you are a physician, you will find the book useful as a tool to help your patients cope with their herpes.

It is my hope that each person reading this book will realize that herpes is everyone's problem and everyone's concern. Whether you think you have herpes or think you don't, you should be armed with the truth when you joke about herpes at a party or when you begin your next intimate relationship. You should know the facts before deciding you never have had or never will have this problem. You should know more than you do now before you agree or disagree that herpes may be "the wrath of God." You must learn more before you decide "it will never happen to me."

This book will give you new insight into a growing problem. It is my hope that the misconceptions which result from ignorance will cease to be the single most important problem about herpes.

1

THE MOST IMPORTANT QUESTIONS FIRST

And you want to travel with her,
you want to travel blind
and you know that she can trust you
because you've touched her perfect body
with your mind.

LEONARD COHEN,
"Suzanne Takes You Down",
Selected Poems, 1956–1968

Am I contagious between recurrences?
Do I have to give up sex?

Medical explanations will be detailed in the forthcoming chapters. For now, remember that **herpes simplex** can exist in two very different states: **active,** in which the virus is growing on the skin, often forming lesions, and **latent,** in which the virus is dormant within the nervous system, causing no harm. The latent period is a quiet period that persists for life. From the latent state the herpes virus may seed a recurrence of an active skin infection.

When your herpes is in the latent state and there is no virus on the skin, your sexual partner cannot be infected. Transmission can only occur when an active skin infection comes into *direct* contact with the skin of another individual. For this reason, people with herpes must learn to carefully avoid sore-to-skin contact when skin lesions are active, resuming normal activity when lesions are not active. Condoms and methods for "safer sex" (see Chapter 12) will add to peace of mind by further reducing the risk of transmission between recurrences. Often, active herpes infections are mild. They are occasionally so mild that nothing is detected. Less often, sores are not detected, yet the herpes is active and can be grown in culture. This makes it imperative for people with herpes to get to know their own recurrence pattern. They can learn to identify the active periods when the virus is on the skin (see Chapter 3) and should acquire the skills necessary for self-examination. They will then adjust their sexual activity patterns around these times, avoiding sore-to-skin contact during the active phases. They must get to know and to understand the facts so that they can inform their partners and explain the risks. Limiting people with herpes to contact with others who have the same infection will accomplish nothing. Furthermore, celibacy will do the world no favor. Indeed, in the long run these extreme efforts will do a great deal of harm, both to the individual person with herpes and to the social acceptance of the disease.

Herpes of the newborn is a deforming, blinding, often fatal disease. Should I give up my plans to have children?

Now that you understand how herpes is spread—from active skin infection and not from latent infection—then you should understand that herpes in a newborn baby (neonatal herpes) may result if the baby is born while the virus is active. This generally occurs if the baby's skin becomes infected during the birth process. If herpes is latent, there is no virus along the birth canal to infect the baby. If herpes sores are present at the time of labor, then (and only then) a cesarean section may be required so that the birth process skips the possibility of direct contact between the infection and the baby. Of course, rupture of the membranes (breaking the bag of waters) is also an important factor because the membranes are a natural barrier for virus traveling up from the mother's skin to the baby's skin. If the membranes rupture and a herpes sore is active, time is of the essence and a cesarean section is performed as an emergency operation. If no sores are present, however, labor may proceed safely and normally.

In order to avoid giving herpes to your baby, you must tell your doctor that you have (or a previous partner had, or your present partner has) herpes. The doctor will then carefully inspect your genital area, especially the external genital area, for herpes sores during labor. You must take an active role and discuss the problem well in advance with your doctor. Regular, careful examinations of the external genitals by your physician during the last two or three weeks of pregnancy are useful. You and the doctor should increase your awareness of your herpes outbreaks—what they feel like, what they look like, and so on. If possible, your doctor will take a herpes "culture" during labor; in the unlikely event that a sore is missed, there will usually be time to watch and treat the baby, if necessary. The chances that a mother with recurrent genital herpes will give birth to a baby who becomes ill with neonatal herpes are only about 1 in 5,000, as long as you and your physician are aware of the status of your infection and are attuned to prevention.

A different syndrome of infection of the fetus may also occur because of herpes infection *inside* the womb. In this situation, herpes could have an adverse effect on the fetus before birth. This syndrome of **congenital herpes** is very rare. Some physicians believe that **primary herpes** (the first episode of herpes) in the mother may lead to womb infection, especially if primary herpes occurs in early pregnancy. There is no hard clinical evidence to support this belief. Indeed, the overwhelming majority of mothers who have primary herpes during pregnancy give birth to perfectly normal babies. Primary herpes in early pregnancy is not considered an "indication" for abortion, although some women in this situation have elected to have an abortion. Nothing specific can be done to prevent congenital herpes, but the risk is very low. In fact, mothers with a proven herpes infection inside the womb have often given birth to completely normal and unaffected babies. It would seem that most healthy and well-nourished babies who were born to women with herpes are very unlikely to develop problems.

When you consider how many new mothers have had a genital herpes infection, it may seem surprising that herpes of the newborn remains an uncommon disease. Some physicians believe that **antibodies** account for this low incidence. Most people with herpes make plenty of herpes antibodies, i.e., proteins that neutralize the virus on contact (see Chapter 2). The antibodies probably get into the amniotic fluid in which the baby floats and coat the baby in a layer of protection. Antibodies may knock out the virus before (or after) it gets to the baby's skin. This is still a theory, but it fits with some of the facts—and the facts are that neonatal herpes is uncommon while genital herpes is common.

I've heard that herpes can cause cancer.
Does that mean it will eventually kill me?

Does herpes infection lead to cancer? The answer here is unknown. Several experiments have been performed which suggest that it *might*. Herpes viruses can "transform" cells in a test tube. This means that, under special rigorous laboratory conditions, the virus can cause a cell that normally reproduces itself poorly or not at all, to live forever—i.e., to change into a "cancer" cell, which reproduces and grows.

Several years ago, investigators noticed that people with more active sex lives had a statistically higher chance of getting cancer of the cervix. Celibacy, then, is one way to avoid cervical cancer. In fact, this cancer almost never occurs in Catholic nuns. If we compare blood samples from women with cervical cancer with blood samples from women with none, we discover that samples from women with cervical cancer are more likely to have herpes antibodies present. Does this prove that herpes caused the cancer—or does it only show that herpes relates to sexual activity and that something else about sexual activity relates to cervical cancer? In fact, there is no question that sex plays a part in the development of cervical cancer. Several investigators believe, however, that it is not herpes—at least not herpes alone—that causes cervical cancer. It could be another sexually transmitted disease such as trichomoniasis or urethritis. Human papillomavirus, which causes genital warts, is now receiving a lot of attention in the area of research into cervical cancer. It appears that certain subtypes of this virus are the main causes of cervical cancer. As the evidence mounts for papillomavirus as a cause, the association between herpes and cervical cancer seems to be rapidly diminishing. Regardless of cause, every woman can take steps to prevent complications of this easily detected cancer.

Happily, cervical cancer is a "good" cancer. It grows very slowly at first and is easy to detect in its early stages. Cure is virtually guaranteed if detected early. Major surgery is generally not required to halt the disease in the early stages. Easy detection is accomplished by the Papanicolaou (Pap) smear, and I recommend one of these regularly for the herpes patient—not only for safety, but also for peace of mind. The Pap test is a quick, simple, and painless test that samples the coating on the cervix (the mouth of the womb). Under the microscope, cancer cells in the specimen can be detected in their earliest stage. This test should be done regularly in all women, but at least once a year in women with herpes. Beyond a regular Pap test, no other precautions against cervical cancer are necessary.

My spouse is my only sexual partner. We've been together for months and I just got herpes. Is my spouse to blame? Has my spouse been unfaithful?

Genital herpes is a sexually transmitted disease. There is a small theoretical possibility of obtaining the infection from another source—for instance, from a warm, moist, shared towel. Practically speaking, however, for the virus to affect the genitals it must be inoculated *onto* the genitals, and the best way of doing that is via sex. But remember that herpes infections come and go, so the virus becomes active, then latent, and then active again. Also, remember that *most* people with genital herpes never have any symptoms that they identify. Your partner could have been infected at some point in the past, yet perhaps it was only recently that you had sex at the exact moment that your partner had an active infection. There is also the possibility that you yourself have had genital herpes for several years and only just now noticed or just started having symptoms. There is no laboratory test that will tell the difference.

Furthermore, if you engage in oral sex, specifically with your partner's mouth in contact with your genitals, then you might get genital herpes because your partner had an active cold sore, or fever blister, or mouth sore (or no recognized symptoms at all), which happened to be caused by herpes. In fact, 50 to 80 percent of us may harbor the virus in a latent state and shed the virus in the mouth during recurrences of active infection. If you have oral sex at the right moment, genital herpes may result. The same virus (herpes simplex) causes both mouth and genital herpes. The mouth type of herpes is usually called **Type 1,** and is most often spread from mouth to mouth (and often from parent to child). Genital herpes is usually called **Type 2.** But herpes simplex is herpes simplex. While Type 1 likes the mouth best and Type 2 likes the genitals best, the virus can be transmitted from one site on one person's body to another site on the partner's body, depending on what body part contacts what. (If the virus is on the toe and if the toe spends a lot of time in someone else's ear, an infection in their ear can result.) So your partner could have received herpes from a parent at age three, have had no symptoms, and still transmit the virus to your genitals 30 years later!

Be careful, then, before calling the divorce lawyer. Talk the problem out with your partner. Don't let herpes alone come between you. Be honest and demand honesty. Possibly your partner was unfaithful and herpes was the first sign—but maybe not. Herpes may, ironically, bring you closer together.

A summary so far

In this chapter we have seen that herpes is able to cause a recurrent skin infection and that often people never realize that they have this infection. However, once herpes has been diagnosed, its recurrence can almost always be clearly recognized by the individual. Avoiding transmission comes naturally once you understand the active phases of infection. Control of your infection comes gradually as your own army of immunity takes over and fights off each recurrence with efficient killing power.

With time, the frequency of recurrences may diminish. The virus may cause a terrible infection in some newborn babies, but it is a highly preventable and uncommon syndrome—and almost always under the control of the mother and her physician if she knows she has herpes and discusses the problem.

A form of cancer may or may not be related to herpes, but it can be easily detected, effectively dealt with, and is unlikely to occur—herpes or no herpes. Is herpes an incurable disease that kills babies and causes cervical cancer? On the contrary, herpes is an extremely common virus infection, poorly understood by many people and further sensationalized by the media. It is a nuisance, without doubt. It *can* be a problem when it recurs very frequently. Safe and effective drug therapy that will reduce the frequency of recurrences is now available. There is no question that herpes can sometimes result in serious complications, but the person who has a herpes infection can easily prevent these complications. Given the right information, herpes is a syndrome that can be under your control.

2
HERPES SIMPLEX: THE VIRUS

We live in a dancing matrix of viruses; they dart, rather like bees, from organism to organism . . . passing around heredity as though at a great party . . . If this is true, the odd virus disease, on which we must focus so much of our attention in medicine, may be looked on as an accident, something dropped.

LEWIS THOMAS,
The Lives of a Cell:
Notes of a Biology Watcher

A short history of herpes

Herpes infections are not new. Over 25 centuries ago Hippocrates, the father of medicine, coined the word "herpes" from the Greek "to creep." Medicine in his time was descriptive. Diseases were classified according to their appearance. In fact, the diseases called "herpes" by this ancient physician are now known to be several different skin maladies with several different names and causes.

During the first part of this century, scientists discovered the "filterable virus," a particle so small that it could pass through a paper filter, so small that it could not be seen with the microscope—yet fully capable of causing infection. It was not long before microbiologists had identified many different viruses capable of causing different diseases. Some examples are polio, hepatitis, influenza, rhinovirus (the common cold), and the herpes viruses. The cause of herpes infections became further understood and the types of viruses further classified.

A great step forward in our understanding of the problem

was developing the technology to grow viruses outside the body, i.e., in the test tube. Since viruses are parasites of cells, the first advance in the field was the discovery that human cells could be stimulated to grow artificially by giving them the right nutrients and salts and keeping them at the right temperature. Cells are the "unit system" of the body. They contain all the parts necessary for reproduction and metabolism; that is, they can make new copies of themselves and eat in between. Furthermore, each type of cell in our body has a special function. It might specialize in movement (muscle cells); structure (bone cells); filtering out poison (kidney cells); detoxification (liver cells); guarding the body surface (epithelial cells); killing foreign invaders (lymphocytes and leukocytes); or carrying oxygen to other cells (erythrocytes).

Pick any organ or functional system of the body—whether it be for pumping blood or for thinking. If you look at a slice of this tissue under the microscope, you will see different cells, each "doing its thing." Figure 1 is from such a slice of normal skin. The cells can be seen lined up according to function, and each cell type has a name: the epithelial cells are the special targets of the herpes simplex virus. Note the thick layer of keratin, a waxy outer coating of skin that forms a natural physical barrier to ward off invasion by infection.

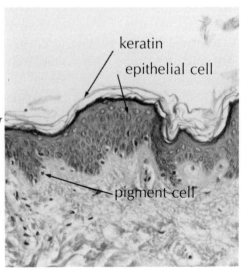

1. A microscope view of a slice of skin. The waxy outer coating of keratin is apparent at the top of the picture. As long as the keratin stays unbroken, it helps to prevent herpes simplex virus from finding its target—the epithelial cells. The cells with the dark pigment (called melanin) give the skin its colour.

Viruses are grown in the laboratory by allowing them to parasitize cells like those from the tissue in Figure 1. First the body cells must be grown in culture. To do this, a piece of tissue is placed in a test tube with chemicals and enzymes and gently chopped up. The separated cells are then given nutrients like sugar, amino acids, and vitamins. If everything goes well, the cells will soon grow and multiply. Figure 2 displays an example of skin cells grown in culture. No longer specialized for skin, these cells are all of the same type, called **fibroblasts**.

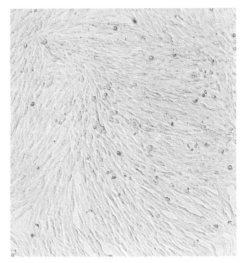

2. Human fibroblast cells grown in tissue culture. This picture is taken through a microscope. Cells in the laboratory look like this if they are healthy —not affected by virus or anything else. Different viruses can be detected by the changes they induce in these cells.

Once scientists were able to grow cells outside the body, getting viruses to do the same inside those cells became easier. Viruses were soon purified, analyzed, and classified. Herpes simplex virus could be detected from sores, on the genitals and elsewhere. At first, herpes was not considered to be a sexually transmitted disease. It was later shown, however, that the greater the number of sexual experiences of an individual, the greater the risk of contracting herpes.

By the late 1960s the syndrome of herpes of the newborn had been analyzed and linked to active herpes infection in the mother at term. This marked the beginning of an explosive period of herpes research. Cervical cancer was connected with herpes. As more became known about the problem, it became more widely publicized, and the public alarm made good press. More people with bothersome sores sought medical help. At the same time, our population became more sexually active. We loosened many of our taboos. Sexual contact often became casual. Oral sexual contact became more frequent. Possibly the most important factor in increasing herpes, however, was the change of birth control methods. As we left behind condoms and foam for the convenience of the IUD and the pill, we left behind these unnatural but effective barriers to infection.

By 1988, we have come up against a reservoir of virus in the community that is so large that herpes has become, literally, almost unavoidable. Today, ten times as many people seek help from a physician for genital herpes as they did ten years ago. You don't have to be a statistician to see the problem we face now and in the future.

What is a virus, anyway?

A virus is a very small living thing. It is so small that it can pass through something as fine as a coffee filter. It cannot live on its own. A virus contains either **DNA** or **RNA** (hereditary material that passes on its characteristics to the next generation of viruses). As shown in Figure 3, this hereditary material is surrounded by a protective outer coat made of protein and sometimes by another protective coat called an **envelope** which is made of fatty and protein-like material.

A virus lives according to all known laws of heredity and natural selection. Its job in life is to reproduce copies of itself. These are called **daughter particles** by virologists. A virus reproduces in a straightforward fashion. First, since it is a parasite, it seeks a host cell that provides a likable environment. Each virus has its own favorite type of host cell. In fact, which cell the virus likes best will partially determine which disease it might cause. For example, hepatitis viruses like liver cells, while herpes simplex viruses like skin and nerve cells.

Figure 4 depicts a herpes infection of an epithelial cell. After finding the cell, the virus makes its presence known by attaching itself (probably to special receptor or receiving sites) to the outer layer of the cell, called the **membrane.** It then undresses itself and injects its hereditary material (DNA or RNA) into the cell. This finds its way to the cell nucleus, where reproduction of new virus daughter particles takes place using the cell's own machinery. Usually this viral reproductive process stops the host cell from living for itself and so, after new virus particles are made, the cell bursts and dies, scattering daughter virus particles around to neighboring cells, where the cycle is repeated. (Note: This was partially abbreviated for clarity.)

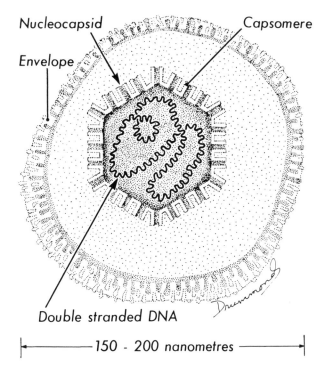

3. This is an artist's drawing of herpes simplex virus. The virus is protected by its envelope, which allows it to attach to cells. The envelope is made of fatty material and is therefore easily dissolved by organic solvents such as alcohol or ether. It is also destroyed by soap. Without the envelope, the virus cannot attach to a cell. The virus core is surrounded by a shell called the capsid. This nucleocapsid consists of 162 subunits called capsomeres, which form a unique geometric shape called an icosahedron. Inside the icosahedral capsid is the double-stranded DNA coiled like a doughnut and weighing in at 100 million daltons. The whole particle measures about 150–200 nanometers (0.0000002 meters) across.

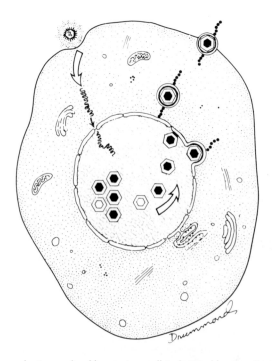

4. *The reproductive cycle of herpes in a cell is depicted by an artist. The virus causing infection finds its way to the epithelial cell surface and attaches to the surface using its envelope (upper left). There it begins the job of reproducing. Reproduction is herpes' role in life. First, after attachment, it injects itself without envelope into the cell, and then the nucleocapsid travels to the nucleus where it injects just its DNA. The DNA makes copies of itself, and these copies fill up newly formed capsids. The filled nucleocapsids pick up new envelopes on their way out of the nucleus and out of the cell itself. (Partially abridged for clarity.)*

    This parasitic relationship of viruses and cells is quite different from bacteria, which can live all on their own. A virus survives by taking over the host cell machinery. That is why it is so hard to kill. Bacteria (like gonorrhea, for example) don't need a host cell to live and grow. They only need basic nutrients (like a good diet with a source of carbohydrates, proteins, and so forth). In fact, it is because bacteria can make so many of their own products that they are so easy to kill with drugs called antibiotics. These substances, such as penicillin, interrupt some manufacturing process which is vital to the bacteria, but of no concern to the human body. The virus needs its host cell, however, and since the virus uses the host cell's manufacturing system for its own life cycle, many chemicals that kill the virus also interrupt the normal host metabolism. That is why, to date, we are without a cure for the common cold—and without a cure for herpes. We are learning more and more about viruses, however. As we find things that viruses do that are unique to the virus, so do we find ways of killing a virus without harming the host.

What stops a viral infection?

This growth cycle of a virus is eventually halted by the coordinated strategy of the body's immune system, which produces specific virus-neutralizing proteins called **antibodies.** These antibodies team up with special infantry fighter cells called **lymphocytes,** and janitor cells called **macrophages.** Antibodies cling to the virus particles and inactivate them. Meanwhile, the lymphocytes kill the few living viruses left over. The macrophages chew up and clean out the mess, leaving room for healthy, unaffected cells to grow and replace the old.

Why don't we develop immunity to herpes? (The story of latent infection)

We really do develop immunity to herpes. In fact, as we've just discussed, this immunity is very effective at stopping a recurrence once it starts. But how, then, is it able to start at all? Herpes simplex has two special tricks up its sleeve to beat the system. Although most of the virus goes through the process just described only to be wiped out by our body's defenses, some virus finds its way up the nerve endings that give feeling to the affected areas of skin.

The body's sensory nervous network is everywhere, giving us feelings, such as pain, temperature sensation, and touch sensation. Nerve fibers extend to all areas of skin like a branching network of phone cables supplying many homes with

phone service. The first switching station is called a **ganglion.**
It gathers up the electrical input from several areas into one
"cable" for transmission to the "central clearing house," the
brain. The ganglia lie next to the spinal cord—the "main
cable"—and house the cell machinery for all those little nerve
fibers. There are several running along the spinal cord from top
to bottom.

The herpes virus stops, as displayed in Figure 5, when it
gets to the ganglion. It comes to rest, for reasons we understand (survival), but by mechanisms we do not understand.
This resting state is so quiet that the body's defenses do not
sense a problem. There is no damage to the nerve, and with no
fight from the body, the virus enters a **latent** state. Exactly

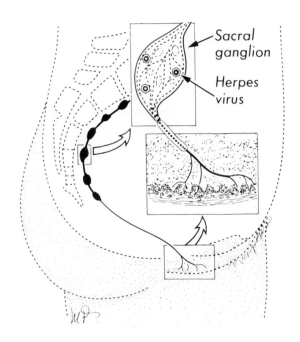

5. During active skin infection, while the infected epithelial cells are going through
their active phases in battle with the immune system, it is thought that the nerve
fibers that supply sensation to the affected areas of skin also become infected (lower
box). The virus travels up the nerve fiber until it gets to the core of the cell inside the
ganglion. There it stops. Unlike the productive and explosive infection occurring on
the skin, infection of the nerve cell results in quiet, or latent, infection that persists
(upper box).

what it is doing in this state is unknown. Some scientists believe that the virus is growing inside the nerve cell but that the infection is slow and "nonproductive." In other words, the virus has entered a state of hibernation where its growth processes slow down. Alternatively, the DNA of the virus may have united with the DNA of the host cell, making them essentially one and the same. Other possibilities certainly exist. There are a couple of facts that are known for sure about latency. First, virus can be cultivated from ganglion cells removed at the time of autopsy under very special conditions of care called **cocultivation.** Second, if a surgeon tampers with a latently infected ganglion, herpes will recur at the original skin site, apparently because tampering reactivates the virus.

For the most part, a latent virus will remain latent. If and when a trigger like a surgeon's scalpel stirs things up, the virus may change its character and decide to reactivate. It will then travel down the same nerve fiber it first went up and will re-enter a healthy skin cell. At this point the active state begins again and a new **recurrent** infection takes place. The recurrent infection once again signals danger to the body's immune system, and those antibodies and cells go to work halting the active infection. This recurrence is often less severe than the first skin infection because neutralizing antibodies were made the first time and are already there, waiting to attack emerging **virions** (daughter virus particles). During the first infection there were no antibodies at first, and so lesions took longer to heal, affected more skin, and caused more blisters and symptoms. Now the immune system is able to halt the recurrence in short order. However, preventing the reactivation from beginning in the first place is not so easy, because the virus is hibernating away in a quiet state, sneaking by the immune system until the process has already reactivated.

Remember, herpes has *two* tricks. The first is its ability to remain latent in the nerve endings. The second is its ability to go from one cell to another without ever leaving the cell environment. Suppose you decided to rob other homes in your neighborhood by going from your house to your neighbor's house without ever going out-of-doors. In that way you could avoid the police. To go a step further, you could send a signal to a carpenter in your neighbor's house telling him to build a self-enclosed bridge until he is inside your house. In fact, this is exactly what herpes simplex virus can do with relatively little effort. The cell with virus can actually fuse with its neighbor cell by inducing bridges. In fact, so many cells may fuse that a **giant cell** is formed. (These giant cells are so specific for herpes that they are one way the virologist can tell if a virus culture is growing herpes.)

Why is this bridging so important? With most viruses, antibodies are sufficient defense to prevent a recurrence. This is, indeed, the basis for preventive vaccines like polio and measles. The vaccine stimulates antibody production: when the virus comes along it is neutralized by the antibodies before it spawns a disease. Since antibody is a very good antivirus poison and since most viruses grow inside cells and then release themselves into the **interstitial** (out-of-doors) environment when the cell bursts, disease cannot recur. Antibodies are waiting, and the infection is nipped in the bud. Herpes is different. Most infected cells do indeed burst, and most virus is indeed neutralized. But antibodies cannot easily travel to the inside of a cell to attack a virus—and herpes is busy building bridges *before* its growth has progressed to the cell-bursting stage. A few virions saunter happily to a neighboring cell, safely protected inside the cell. Other emerging young virions will be killed effectively in a few hours when they break outside, but a select few live on and infect healthy neighboring cells. Quite a trick! Of course, the immune system cuts this process off by using its lymphocytes and macrophages—just as our imaginary scheme for robbing houses would not get very far before the police put a stop to it.

We can now understand why antibodies are helpful in limiting the severity of recurrent disease, yet useless in preventing the recurrence entirely. Herpes is very effective at hiding from its enemies. Hippocrates chose a remarkably apt name—"to creep."

What is a herpes virus?

The herpes family of viruses includes five different viruses which affect human beings:

1. **Epstein-Barr virus** is the major cause of mono—**infectious mononucleosis** ("kissing disease").
2. **Cytomegalovirus** may also cause mono. It may also be sexually transmitted and may cause problems to newborns. It can cause hepatitis. Occasionally it is transmitted by blood transfusion. It is very common among homosexual men and is associated with (but not the cause of) **AIDS**, or the **acquired immune deficiency syndrome** we are hearing so much about. We have a lot to learn about this virus.
3. **Herpes zoster** (also called **Varicella zoster**) is the cause of chickenpox. Chickenpox is the primary (first-time) infection. This virus may also recur. The recurrent form is commonly known as **shingles.**
4. **Herpes simplex virus Types 1 and 2** is the subject of this book. Depending on the situation, it may cause *cold sores* or *genital herpes*, or, less commonly, *herpes of the newborn* and *herpes encephalitis*.
5. **Human herpes virus Type 6** is a newly observed agent found in the blood cells (T lymphocytes) of a few patients with a variety of diseases affecting the immune system. Little else is known about this new virus since studies are just beginning.

These five viruses are similar in that they are large viruses. Their hereditary material is double-stranded DNA. Each has a protective envelope. Under the electron microscope, herpes viruses cannot be differentiated. Each of the first four types remains latent for life. We do not yet know about the fifth. Of these four types, most people in the world have acquired all of them by adulthood, and most will tend to recur from time to time. Yet in a similar way to the latent state of herpes simplex virus, each of these viruses does no harm during latency. Latency is *not* a disease. Recurrences of active infection may cause symptoms, however. For example, the elderly gentleman with a painful bout of shingles is having a recurrence of a virus infection called chickenpox, which he first caught in early childhood. For 80 years he has harbored the latent herpes zoster virus in his ganglia; the virus left him unaffected for 80 years until an active recurrence took place.

Here the similarities end, however. These different herpes viruses do not cause the same diseases. Infection with one does *not* make infection with another more likely. Nor does infection with one *prevent* infection with another.

Yes, your grandmother with shingles has "herpes," but because of its notoriety, the word "herpes" has come to mean *herpes simplex*, one of the five members of the human herpes viruses.

3

GENITAL HERPES: THE SYMPTOMS

Yes, it is the exact location of the soul that I am after. The smell of it is in my nostrils. I have caught glimpses of it in the body diseased. If only I could tell it. Is there no mathematical equation that can guide me? So much pain and pus equals so much truth?
RICHARD SELZER,
Mortal Lessons:
Notes on the Art of Surgery

What are the symptoms of genital herpes?

Any infection may cause a spectrum of disease symptoms from very mild to very severe. Herpes is no different. In other words, there are some people who suffer no symptoms whatsoever from the infection who can be proven by some lab test to have had infection, while, on the other hand, there are people whose symptoms are so severe that they may result in severe disability or even death. An example of the latter would be a newborn baby who becomes infected with herpes that disseminates throughout the body.

When it causes infection in a normal person, however, genital herpes almost never causes disease at the far end of the spectrum; that is, it almost never results in severe disability or death. In fact, the majority of people with genital herpes find themselves at the opposite end of the spectrum. They have been exposed to genital herpes, developed latent infections and antibodies, but deny ever having had symptoms of this infection! It is difficult, then, to paint any single picture of what a herpes infection is like. The symptoms depend not only on the severity of infection, but also on the site of the infection. The site of initial infection is largely determined by the site of in-oculation. In other words, where did the herpes virus find its easiest access to epithelial cells of the skin? For the most part, herpes simplex likes mucous membranes. Mucous membranes are areas where the skin is thin. These include areas like the labia (lips) of the vagina and the lips of the mouth. However, any area of the body may be fair territory for herpes. If a finger has a tiny crack (which it commonly does), any herpes simplex virus sitting on the finger could easily find its way to an epithelial cell. In general, though, the virus will avoid places like the hand and other thick-skinned areas because in these places it is more difficult for the virus to find its way in. How-ever, any time there is excessive moisture and especially if there is trauma or injury that compromises the normal protec-tion of the area, the setting is ideal for herpes to be trans-mitted.

With genital herpes there are three major classifications of outbreaks: **primary** infection; **nonprimary initial** infection; and **recurrent** infection.

Primary infection

The person who experiences a true primary infection has never previously been exposed to any herpes simplex virus at any time. In other words, there is no history of cold sores, there is no history of exposure to cold sores, and this person has devel-oped no previous antibodies to herpes. The absence of antibodies is crucial. Antibodies, remember, are capable of neutralizing herpes virus quite effectively. The body, in defense of its first attack by virus, has the job of making antibodies. It usually does so quite effectively. Once antibodies are present, herpes infections become very different.

During this first (primary) infection, however, the virus can be inoculated, or transferred, to surrounding areas of skin. In-fection may be much more severe because no antibodies are yet present. More sores may develop. In addition, there is a greater chance that a person will feel generally sick with his or her primary infection. Usually this is a flu-like illness. It feels very much like any other viral infection causing muscle aches and pains, and possibly fever and headaches. Primary infection, however, causes a spectrum of disease symptoms. In other words, for some people primary infection may pass unnoticed with only a bit of vaginal discharge or even without a hint of a problem.

When genital sores erupt, they generally do so at the site of inoculation, which is usually on the external genitals. Sores will generally look like a cluster of small blisters filled with clear or whitish fluid. The classical herpes sore, seen in Figure 6, is just this: a group of small blisters —**vesicles** —on a red base of inflamed skin.

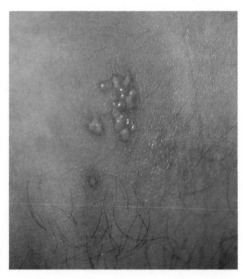

6. A picture of a typical or classical recurrence of skin herpes. A cluster of fluid-filled vesicles is seen overlying a red base of inflamed skin. These sores are itchy and may be somewhat painful, especially if touched directly.

Often these blisters are never seen, and the first signs of infection are small erosions of the skin called **ulcers.** Ulcers also tend to come in clusters, or groups.

In women, herpes sores or lesions are usually on the external genitalia, most commonly on the labia of the vagina. Another common site is the area covered by pubic hair. In men, sores are usually on the foreskin or shaft of the penis or in the

pubic area, but the glans (tip) of the penis is also possible territory. More than one of these areas may be affected during primary herpes. Sores may vary in size from very small (one to
two millimetres) to very large (one to two centimetres). Sores
are usually quite superficial, with the infection on the out-
ermost layer of the skin. The skin becomes raw and painful and
itchiness is the rule. There is a lot of inflammation going on at
this time because the body is attacking the virus. This is a
healthy response, but may lead to quite a bit of distress. If
sores are present around the **urethral meatus,** the spot for
exit of urine, urination may become quite uncomfortable.
People may complain of **external dysuria**, or the feeling that
urine stings once it has exited and has touched the sores. Sores
might also appear on the thighs, on the buttocks, or around the
anus. In addition, sores may be present in other areas, for example, the mouth. If oral contact occurred with the same area
as genital contact, there is a possibility that a mouth infection
might result. Rare sites of infection, and again depending upon
the place of virus inoculation, will be the fingers, the breasts,
or the eyes.

Often the lymph nodes are swollen in the **inguinal**, or
groin, region. This means that the immune system is fighting
off the virus. **Lymph nodes** are those "glands" that the doctor
often feels for in the neck when you have a cold. Similar
"glands" are present throughout the body. Those in the groin
(see Figure 7) are the areas of lymph drainage from the genital
area. With genital infection these groin lymph nodes may become swollen and tender to the touch since the lymph system
is an important component of the body's immune system.

The outer portion of the urinary tract itself may become infected with herpes, resulting in discomfort on urination or even
difficulty in passing urine. Internally, the cervix (the mouth of
the womb) is infected about 80 to 90 percent of the time during
primary infection. Except for the vaginal discharge, cervical infection causes little in the way of symptoms. Occasionally the
doctor can see herpes sores on the cervix. However, during
primary herpes, some herpes virus is usually on the cervix,
whether there are sores to be seen or not. Infection of the

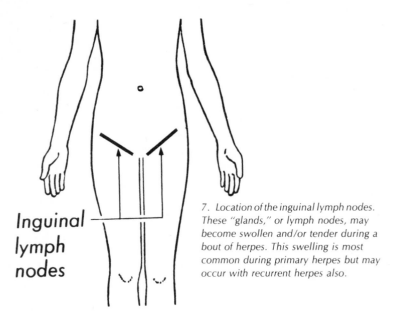

Inguinal lymph nodes

7. Location of the inguinal lymph nodes. These "glands," or lymph nodes, may become swollen and/or tender during a bout of herpes. This swelling is most common during primary herpes but may occur with recurrent herpes also.

cervix may cause a runny vaginal discharge. However, when an unusual vaginal discharge is present, it may be caused either by herpes or by some other infection going on at the same time. Discharge may also be a normal phenomenon. If a discharge is present, it is important to find out if some other cause such as trichomoniasis or a yeast infection is present *along with* the herpes. In fact, whether or not discharge is present, a physician or a specially trained paramedical person must examine you for other treatable infections that may occur at the same time as herpes.

So, as you can see, primary herpes infections may cause anything from no symptoms to painful sores, from a sore throat to headache and muscle pains. It can cause any or all of these symptoms. Symptoms will clear up and disappear completely, usually within two to three weeks. Occasionally people complain that they didn't feel quite right for several weeks after their primary infection. There is no good explanation for this feeling, but it is a common complaint. The ulcer-like sores will eventually scab over and these dry crusts will fall off. This will mark the end of the primary infection.

Nonprimary initial infection

Nonprimary initial infection means that this is the first episode of *symptoms* of herpes. However, the person with nonprimary initial herpes has an "immune memory" for herpes simplex virus. This may result from previous infection with herpes simplex Type 1 or Type 2. Remember, that 50 to 80 percent of people have some antibodies to herpes simplex virus, usually because they were exposed to someone's cold sores in childhood or because of a primary genital infection that gave no symptoms. So, in fact, the first infection with herpes is commonly of the nonprimary variety. Nonprimary initial herpes is very different from primary herpes because of the immune system. These antibodies, lymphocytes, etc., which have already "learned" about herpes, are ready to be quickly triggered. Since there is already a mechanism built in to fight this infection, the body combats the disease effectively and rapidly. The symptoms are essentially the same as for recurrent herpes. It has a special name only because it is the first episode to be noticed. The sexual contact which resulted in transmission of this nonprimary initial episode of infection may have been recent, or may have occurred months, or even years, before the onset of symptoms.

Recurrent infection

Recurrent herpes is usually much milder than primary. Again, symptoms are the result of herpes infections of epithelial (skin) cells. However, recurrent infection begins when virus is inoculated into these cells by traveling back down the nerve pathway that it originally traveled up on its way to creating latent infection of the ganglion (see Figure 5, page 31). This time there are antibodies present and an "immune memory"; that is, the body has seen the herpes virus before and is quite effective at limiting its growth.

In fact, people with recurrent herpes are often troubled very little in terms of their physical ailments during recurrences. Sores are usually limited to a few. They may be single or multiple, and they tend to come in clusters, often grouped together on a small, reddened, inflamed base of skin. Recurrences will often begin with some sensation or warning sign that something is wrong, for example, a pain in the leg, or tingling or itching in one area of the genitals. The warning sign may be present for anywhere from a few minutes to a few days. If the area affected is usually an area of dry skin (for example the buttocks, thigh, or penile shaft), then sores may develop first as tiny blisters (also called vesicles). Blisters are filled with clear or whitish fluid and are usually grouped together on a red base of skin. The vesicles soon turn into wet skin erosions, or ulcers. On areas of wet skin (labia of the vagina or under the foreskin of the penis) this may happen so quickly that the actual blister is never noticed. In other words, the first physical sign would be an ulcer. The ulcer will then often scab over with a dry crust, which soon falls off. Unlike primary infection, this recurrent herpes sequence usually takes just a few days from start to finish. Fewer lesions develop, less virus is present, and the discomfort is much less. Itchiness is common. Although variable, the sores are usually tender to touch directly, but they may not hurt a great deal if left alone. If, however, the sores are in a place where they are hit by urine or rubbed, pain may be more prominent. That general feeling of sickness that comes with primary infection is usually absent. Sores are in the same places as discussed in primary herpes, except that the cervix is usually not affected. In other words, genital herpes is an affliction, generally, of the external genitals (the parts you can see with your clothes off, holding a mirror and a light). The internal genitals are usually not affected during recurrences.

As with primary herpes, the symptoms of recurrent herpes will depend upon the area affected. Generally, one small area of one of the sites pictured in Figure 8 will be affected during one recurrence. The site may stay precisely the same at each recurrence for some people. It may be slightly different each time for another. It might hurt when it occurs in one site but itch in another.

It is important to reiterate the wide range of severity here.

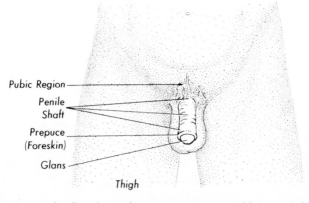

Pubic Region

Penile
Shaft

Prepuce
(Foreskin)

Glans

Thigh

8 A. Commonly affected genital areas in recurrent genital herpes —male.

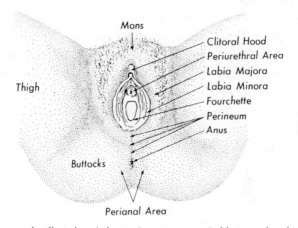

Mons

Clitoral Hood
Periurethral Area
Labia Majora
Labia Minora
Fourchette
Perineum
Anus

Thigh

Buttocks

Perianal Area

8 B. Commonly affected genital areas in recurrent genital herpes —female.

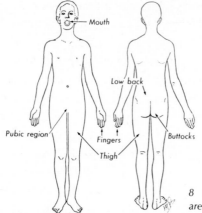

Mouth

Low back

Pubic region   Fingers   Buttocks

Thigh

8 C. Commonly affected nongenital areas in "genital" herpes.

43

Active recurrent sores may be obviously herpes when they come in clusters of little blisters. But genital herpes may never be more severe than one very small sore on the labia or foreskin or around the anus or on the thigh. It may be the size of a pencil eraser or it may be as small as the sharpened lead point. The sore may, in fact, never be painful at all in some people. It may not even itch! This means that it is necessary to heighten your awareness that herpes is variable. Realize that it may hurt over here but itch over there. Assume that any break in the skin in an area depicted in Figure 8 is herpes unless you know otherwise. Use a mirror to look and a wet finger to rub lightly over the areas, looking for tender or red or swollen spots that might be active herpes. Get to know your herpes and anything else of an unusual nature happening on your genitals. On the other hand, try not to be obsessed about it. You need to know if you're having herpes when you're planning to have sex. If you are having only minor skin problems or discomfort much of the time, which only rarely turn into a classical herpes sore, then there could well be some other explanation for the sensations you're having or the skin breaks you're noticing. For example, you might be having a bacterial or a yeast vaginal infection or you might be confused about what is a sore and what is not.

On the other side of the coin, getting too cavalier about genital discomfort is not good either. People commonly get herpes and other things confused, especially before they get to know their herpes. Herpes will often be misidentified as a spider bite (especially on the leg or the buttocks—see Figure 9); yeast infection (see Figure 10); hemorrhoid; pimples (on the buttocks, labia, etc.); shingles; water blisters; cuts or slits of the vagina or lips; soreness from vigorous sex.

The appearance and sequence of herpes sores are discussed in the coming pages. With each description, however, this spectrum of variable severity must be kept in mind. The phases might all occur in the obvious sequence. They can last a week or an hour. Some phases can be skipped. Rarely, a person may need a hospital bed to recover from herpes. Someone in this situation will usually know the diagnosis! Others will never notice anything unusual. It will become possible for you to reach a happy medium of good awareness of your body without being concerned over unrelated twinges. Achieving this happy medium may take a few months, but it will come. When herpes phases are inactive, there is generally no virus on the skin, so no symptoms occur and transmission of infection does not take place. In any one person, an active recurrence may occur never, once in a lifetime, once in a year, or as often as three to four times a month.

What are the phases of herpes infections?

The phases are very important to learn because they determine when the living virus is on the skin. An active infection may be categorized as: **asymptomatic; prodrome** (warning); **early redness; vesicles; wet ulcers; crusts; healed.**

During the **asymptomatic** phase, the virus is latent. Residing in the ganglion, it causes absolutely no harm. It is not on the skin. If you know what herpes feels like and know what it looks like (and you've looked and found none), you can be nearly sure that no virus is there. (See Chapter 5 for further details on transmission.) Herpes cannot jump from your ganglion to the genitals of your sexual partner. It is only passed on when it is active on the skin. You can do a great deal to prevent this transmission if you know what is active, you've looked carefully for herpes sores, and you've checked out any unusual feelings in the common areas of infection.

Furthermore, if virus is causing no symptoms but is active, the amount of virus should be very small. Let us say that for some reason you missed an active herpes because you just could not see it or feel it. You have had sexual contact anyway. Since there probably is an "inoculating dose," that is, a minimum number of virus particles that must be contacted in order to get herpes, this period is probably still a low-risk phase for transmitting the infection.

Most people who get recurrent herpes (but not all) will have a **prodrome** or warning. This signifies that the virus has been reactivated and is on its way to the skin. As the virus activates, the nerve may react and symptoms may develop. The warning is different for everyone. In some it will be a pain in the leg or the buttocks. In others a feeling of numbness or coldness or itching or pain may develop right at the spot where the sores are soon going to appear. The most common prodromal is this itching at the site before the lesions appear. Occasionally, herpes starts with a special kind of headache or a fever. This prodromal phase may last five minutes or three days. Most commonly, it goes on for about 12 to 24 hours. It may be something you've never noticed. It is a good thing to think about and identify this phase in yourself, if possible. It tells you that the active sequence has started. At this time some people will begin to have a virus present on the skin. Skin contact with geni-

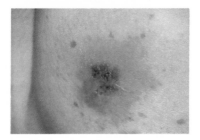

9. Herpes on the buttock is commonly much larger, often more uncomfortable, and usually longer lasting than outbreaks on the genital area. These outbreaks are actually manifestations of recurrent genital herpes appearing on the buttocks, but they are commonly misdiagnosed as shingles or spider bites.

tal areas or other areas where you usually get sores should stop until this recurrence is over. It is very common for this phase to come and go, often without other phases following. Many people realize that they have had a warning after it is over. In other words, there will be a vague sensation, below the level of consciousness, that something is amiss. Once a sore is there, there is the recognition, "Oh yeah, I felt that all day." This requires back-stepping in your mind. If you have warnings, try to notice them as they occur. They will help you to learn to map out these active phases of infection. If you have

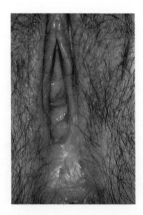

10. The extensive redness and ulceration seen here was confused with a bad outbreak of herpes. The patient's predominant symptom was itching. Cultures showed yeast. She was easily treated for that and felt fine in a couple of days.

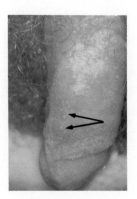

11 A. A picture of a sore in the vesicle stage. These fluid-filled, tiny blisters often come in clusters, but they may come one at a time. The fluid can be clear, white, or red.

no warnings, then your active phases of infection begin with the development of a lesion.

Next, **early redness** may be detected in a small area of skin. It may feel itchy or painful to the touch, or just sensitive. At this point, virus is beginning to grow inside the skin (epithelial) cells. The immune system of antibodies and lymphocytes is being called back to work. The ensuing battle between defenses and virus causes inflammation or redness. Virus is in the skin. Contact with the area where a sore is developing is unwise.

Vesicles are the small blisters that form on top of the early red patch. They have clear or whitish fluid (see Figure 11A). There may be only one vesicle, or they may be in groups, with only a few or with so many that they run together. The tops of these blisters are very thin and come off easily, often oozing a little of the fluid. The fluid is the product of the sick, swollen skin cells that have been attacked by herpes. As the inflammation continues, itchiness and/or pain is often, but not universally, present. Virus is virtually *always* present at this stage, making this a good time for getting a culture diagnosis. This stage is commonly skipped, especially in women with labial sores and men with sores under the foreskin, since these wet areas quickly macerate the blister and rub off its top, leaving an ulcer underneath. In fact, just touching these vesicles may cause them to break and leak fluid. A vesicle poked with a cotton swap or the tip of your finger will be quite tender, even if it is not bothersome just sitting there. Avoid breaking vesicles on purpose, however, since there is nothing to be gained by doing this.

The next phase is characterized by **wet ulcers**, which are really the vesicles with their tops off. Several examples can be seen in Figure 11B. They glisten with wetness and may feel raw to the touch. There may be one tiny sore that can only be seen with a magnifying lens, or there may a dozen large and tender ulcers. They may group together to form larger ulcers. Herpes ulcers are superficial; that is, they are right at the skin surface. They are not deep and ragged but tend to be rather round and wet. Tender to the touch is the rule, but there are exceptions. Virus is virtually *always* present at this point also. From as far away as the eye, wet ulcers may look like a small cut or a red, swollen area. Spread away the pubic hair, if necessary, for a good look. Use a magnified mirror. If you can, touch the sore with a cotton swab or a wet finger again to see if it is tender.

When the fluid in the ulcers begins to dry, the sores cover themselves with a **dry crust,** or scab. Examples are shown in Figure 11C. This phase marks the beginning of healing and virus begins to disappear. The scab covers the raw ulcer just as a scab grows over a cut from a knife. At first the scab may be soft and wet and crumbly. If rubbed away, a wet ulcer remains underneath. As the sore dries, however, the crust hardens. Underneath the skin grows anew. This is called re-epithelialization. While the crust is still there, virus may be present. Sexual contact within the area of the sore is still not advisable. The itch or pain may be leaving entirely, or the itch might just begin to worsen at this stage. The size of the lesion will generally determine the size of the scab. Commonly, small sores never have a crust stage. They just seem to melt away from ulcer to nothing. Others always get a dry crust.

The sores are **healed** when the crust falls off and the active infection is over. This is the same as the asymptomatic phase. The healing may leave a residual red mark (Figure 12A), just like a healed cut from a knife. These spots may also be whitish (Figure 12B) rather than red, or they may in some other way appear different from the unaffected skin. The marks may be slightly tender, but the surface is definitely healed with new skin. This skin is smooth and knit back together and feels normal to the touch. The visible mark may last for weeks, or it may be present for only a few days. Some people will never get marks. Virus growth is over; only healing is active. Skin contact with this area is now safe once again. This healed phase generally occurs five to ten days after the appearance of the vesicle stage in recurrent herpes. However, the time may be measured in hours, or occasionally (rarely) in weeks. During primary herpes, however, the "natural history" of a single outbreak is quite a bit longer (approximately three weeks).

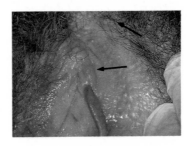

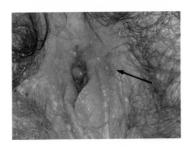

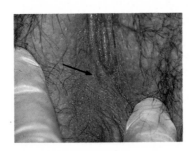

11 B. Herpes sores in the wet ulcer stage.

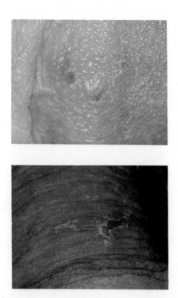

11 C. Herpes sores in the crusted stage. Crusts can be wet or dry.

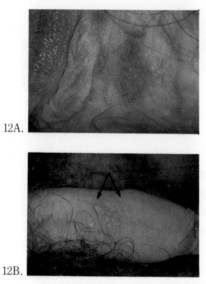

12. Pictures of herpes sores in the healed phase. After healing, skin may appear totally normal or
A. healed sores might have increased colour, or
B. decreased colour.
These colour changes can persist for weeks or even months. They do not mean that herpes is active. This is an inactive phase.

Remember that not every phase occurs in every person. One or several of the phases may be skipped. For example, warnings may occur and no sores develop. Ulcers may develop with no warning or blisters. Ulcers may heal with no crust stage. The stages are still important, however. Put simply, when no symptoms are present and when no sores are visible (and you've looked), or when only residual redness is left, the active infection is over.

What are the trigger factors?

Several studies suggest that latent herpes may reactivate because of trigger factors. These factors are poorly understood, however, and are for the most part unavoidable. The known trigger factors include: the menstrual cycle; emotional stress; another illness, especially with fever; sexual intercourse; surgery; injury; sunlight; and certain medications.

Every person's trigger factor is different. For example, while many women will get herpes only during a certain part of the menstrual cycle, the trigger day of the cycle varies from woman to woman. One study suggests that more women develop recurrences 5 to 12 days before the onset of their next menstrual period than at other times. Unfortunately, birth control pills, which stop the normal cycling hormones, don't seem to diminish recurrences, but careful studies have not been performed.

Emotional stress may be important for some, but for others stress is unrelated to herpes outbreaks. I find that trying to force away stress in an attempt to rid onself of herpes might succeed in making a lot of new stress. In fact, no one has ever proven that stress causes herpes to recur. Since herpes itself is stressful, how can we be sure which is the "chicken" and which is the "egg"? This is a virus infection, not an episode of the jitters. Reactivation of latent infection in the nervous system is a very complex problem that remains poorly understood. Easy answers to tough questions like control of "triggers" may be misleading and create false hopes. That is not to say that getting rid of stress is not a good idea. Many people strongly believe that stress control can lead to herpes control. Indeed, a sizeable proportion of persons who have herpes relate their outbreaks to stress. It is difficult to give general advice. I encourage anyone to take steps to reduce life's stresses. On the other hand, I encourage everyone to avoid feeling a sense of failure or guilt if efforts at stress control do not reduce herpes outbreaks.

Some people say that sexual intercourse leads to sores. This is also a tough one. Most times I find that these are healed sores, usually in the residual redness phase, that have a very thin layer of skin over them that tears easily during intercourse. This occurs mainly in people who have very frequent recurrences. They resume sex after healing, only to find a new sore in the morning. This is frustrating, indeed, but probably sex is not the trigger. Rather, sex is the innocent victim of unfortunate circumstance. If you feel that sex triggers recurrences, try waiting a few extra days after healing before resuming sexual contact. It may be the abrasion itself. Try slow and gentle sex and lubricants. Make sure that this really is herpes, by returning to your physician with a new sore. Depending on your individual situation, oral acyclovir may have a role to play here (see Chapter 11).

Surgery and injury are just unavoidable. Sunlight is avoided by covering affected areas with clothing or commercial sunblocking agents. Dr. S. Spruance from the University of Utah recently presented intriguing data on the use of oral acyclovir in patients who were prone to developing sunlight-triggered cold sores. He treated them effectively, before they developed symptoms at all, by predicting that their cold sores would develop after skiing. He went to the ski slopes to get his volunteers. Oral acyclovir, of course, is extremely effective at prevention (see Chapter 11), much more effective than when it is used after the beginning of even the earliest symptoms of infection. Now if we could figure out all the triggers in advance of recurrence onset, this drug could be taken intermittently to prevent disease. Thus far, however, the only trigger with this predictability level is sunlight on the lip.

As far as medications go, make sure you need pills before

you take them. That includes megavitamins. Never use cortisone creams or any of the derivatives of cortisone (ask your doctor or pharmacist) to treat herpes. If they must be used for another reason, make sure the reason is a good one. Nothing will help a herpes virus live a long, healthy, active life like cortisone will. In fact, any ointment other than specific antiviral medication may prolong the duration of sores.

If I've had a first episode of herpes, will I get a recurrence?

There is no way to predict who will get a recurrence and who will not. Most people will have at least a few. If your herpes simplex virus is a Type 2 (as opposed to Type 1) you will be more likely to have recurrences. A recent report by Dr. Corey's group at the University of Washington suggests that 84 percent of women and 100 percent of men who have first episodes of genital herpes get at least one recurrence. For some people, recurrences get milder and less frequent with time, although you should not keep a calendar and expect each recurrence to be shorter than the last. Indeed, these studies suggest that there may be no specific reduction in the frequency of episodes over the first two years. Basically, the recurrence pattern and severity vary a lot. In fact, if there is one thing you can be sure of, it is that the recurrence pattern will change from time to time. Overall, the average number of recurrences is about four per year.

Recurrences of herpes can start even as the primary infection heals. Recurrences may come one on top of the other, so one may begin as another is ending. They may occur once on the labia and next on the thigh, or always in the same place. No treatment during the initial episode has yet been devised that will affect the pattern of future recurrences. The reasons for differences in recurrence patterns are poorly understood. Some people only get recurrences. In other words, their first symptoms occur months or years after their last sexual contact. The first infection was so mild that no symptoms occurred, yet latent infection was established. Something later triggered the recurrence.

Can I have herpes without any symptoms?

Several studies have shown that antibody directed against herpes can be detected very frequently in the blood. Similarly, herpes can be found in the sacral ganglia of autopsy cases. Many of these people have no history whatsoever of genital herpes. Furthermore, about half of the people with herpes have not had any contact with a person with herpes that they know of. Even in a private room with a physician listing symptoms, people who have had sexual contact with someone who has primary genital herpes very often deny any symptoms of herpes. This is not because they are lying. Rather, it reflects the fact that herpes commonly causes no symptoms.

The explanation for this is not clear. However, it is easy to see how a mild herpes blister, looking like a pimple or a tiny pinhole, might go unnoticed. Even a really severe infection on the cervix, if localized to the cervix or other internal genital area, may cause no symptoms whatsoever. An infinite number of scenarios to explain innocent transmission may be imagined. For example, a recurrent sore around the anus may cause recurrent rectal itching. This is a symptom which nearly everyone has at one time or another and could easily be passed off as insignificant. Can anyone honestly deny ever having had an itch in the rectum?

Must herpes always hurt?

No. Herpes sores often do not hurt. Even though we have heard elsewhere of stories of terrible pain, these more severe symptoms are most prominent during the primary infection. Sores that are open and raw are commonly tender and painful to touch. Push a cotton swab on a sore and it will hurt. Urinate on a sore and it will hurt. Itching may be more common than pain during recurrences, however. Pain is a funny thing. People sense pain differently.

Some people with recurrent herpes never feel anything and only know they are active by looking at the sores. Others are exquisitely aware of the slightest change in their body's chemistry. Regardless, pain is usually not the major problem in coping with recurrent herpes.

On the other hand, patients with strong primary infections may suffer extreme pain for a short time. It may be too painful to urinate, to sit, or to walk. Hospitalization with intravenous therapy and painkillers may be required. It can be very frightening to imagine this pain recurring every month for a lifetime. Happily it does not. If you are reading this during your primary, remember that herpes may recur, but it will never again do what it is doing now. Recurrent herpes is not a recurrence of primary herpes. It is generally much milder. Sores are smaller and less painful and are usually gone after several days. The virus does not make you sick as it might have done during primary herpes.

Can herpes cause other kinds of pain?

Because herpes likes nerves, it may cause irritation of the nerves. During reactivation (the prodrome phase) the virus is traveling down the nerve and may cause pain in other areas where the nerve runs. This pain is often in the leg or buttocks and is called a **sacral paresthesia.** It usually disappears when the prodrome phase is over. Headache may also be a warning sign. A rare patient will get reactivation of the virus traveling *up* the nerve instead of down; that is, the virus gets into the central nervous system and causes meningitis, or an inflammation of the sac around the brain. This is not harmful. It does not damage the nervous system, but if it happens it is quite distressing and results in headache, stiff neck, aversion to bright lights, and fever. It does get better. If this occurs, seek the care of a physician so that you can be sure it is just herpes. (Other causes of meningitis may require specific therapy.) An unusual, but not rare, complaint after an active recurrence is residual pain in the area involved. The skin might be painful or prickly, or it may feel as if it is drawn too tightly. Generally this complaint fades with time. It is called **postherpetic neuralgia.** Postherpetic neuralgia happens very commonly following a herpes zoster skin infection (shingles). Note that it *follows* active infection and, therefore, does not represent active virus shedding. It would be an inactive phase. Happily, this is not usually a sequel to a bout of herpes simplex.

Can herpes make me sterile?

No, but a number of other sexually transmitted infections can cause sterility, for example, **gonorrhea** and **Chlamydia.** These other infections are treatable. The most common warning signs are urethral (male) or vaginal (female) discharge, painful urination, or a painful lower abdomen. These internal genital infections can cause enough inflammation around the ovaries and tubes in a woman to result in scarring, making it difficult for the egg to reach the womb. This may cause sterility. A culture test and examination for pus cells will generally detect these internal genital infections. Many people, both male and female, have no symptoms of these other infections, whatsoever. The doctor who diagnoses herpes should also test for these infections, especially since they are easy to cure with certain antibiotics. In addition, herpes may be confused with **syphilis** and other diseases even by the most expert, most widely experienced physician. Only laboratory tests can distinguish the different sexually transmitted infections with 100 percent accuracy. Make sure you undergo these tests at least once.

Can herpes make me impotent?

Impotence means that a man is unable to obtain and sustain an erection when he feels like doing so. Herpes often has a detrimental effect on feeling like it, especially during the period of anger after acquiring herpes. Anger, as well as depression and other emotional factors, may commonly influence sexual urges in men and women with herpes. Usually such changes in urges are related to correctable things, such as getting over the fear of talking herpes over with your partner. Changes in sexual urges are normal and common. They should not stay for a long time.

Impotence is often based on emotional factors as well. Most times true impotence results from similar feelings that might potentially diminish sexual urges, such as anger or the feeling of having an "incurable" infection. Severe primary herpes infections of males, especially homosexual males with proctitis (rectal-anal infection), may uncommonly result in physical impotence as a result of nerve inflammation. This inflammation leaves after the acute infection and generally does not recur. There are other more common physical causes for impotence, however, such as diabetes mellitus, certain drugs, and hormonal imbalances. If impotence or loss of sexual desire is sustained, you should seek specific medical attention for the problem.

Are cold sores (fever blisters) also herpes?

Yes, for the most part, fever blisters are caused by herpes simplex. The virus is usually (but not always) Type 1. Sores generally look like genital herpes, but they occur on the lip or the skin near the lip. Mouth herpes—like genital herpes—is most often an external disease. The classic cold sore occurs at the vermilion border of the lip—the point where the thin mucous membrane of the mouth changes abruptly into the skin of the face (the outer edge of the lipstick). Ulcers in the side of the mouth may be herpes, but usually these are **aphthous ulcers,** which are not infectious. Cracks in the corners of the mouth are usually not caused by herpes.

True cold sores go through a similar sequence of active phases as already described. The ganglion for latency with the cold sore is called the trigeminal ganglion. It is located inside the skull. In fact, the mouth is the most common site for herpes recurrences. Sounds like genital herpes is a bit like a cold sore of the genitals? That's almost exactly correct. In fact, a person with mouth herpes can give a sexual partner genital herpes by having direct oral-to-genital contact while oral infection is active. The nature of herpes sores and the sites affected are largely dependent upon what gets inoculated where.

Can I have received my infection months, or even years, before my first symptoms?

Yes. Primary herpes is usually, but not necessarily, quite uncomfortable. Remember that herpes infections form a spectrum from no symptoms to severe symptoms. Initial infection may pass unnoticed. At a later date recurrent herpes that does cause symptoms may begin.

A true primary infection, however, with its accompanying pain, numerous lesions, fever, etc., is unlikely to have been caused by a remote infection. The incubation period for primary herpes is probably between 2 and 30 days in general, and it is then that primary infection occurs. If your first outbreak is mild, this could be a nonprimary, initial infection. It could be the first recurrence after an asymptomatic primary infection that took place weeks, months, or even years before. In this case, the incubation period is more difficult to pinpoint with certainty. If properly performed during the first episode, an antibody test will separate the primary from the nonprimary initial infection. If you have a positive test showing antibodies (nonprimary), however, you still will not know if the infection was just received from recent contact (and you already had antibody), or if it was long ago received from remote contact (you developed antibody then) with newly established symptoms. Drs. Bernstein, Lovett, and Bryson from UCLA recently reported that 17 of 24 individuals experiencing nonprimary initial genital herpes had pre-existing antibodies to herpes simplex Type 2. This would suggest that some may have been experiencing their first symptoms of a process that first began with transmission at a much earlier date.

I often get prodromal symptoms, but no sores. What does that mean?

Warning signs without sores probably means reactivation. Most people who get warning symptoms with sores will also get them without sores. This means that the virus has reactivated. It may have traveled to the skin, but, in some way, the body has stopped the infection before it could cause sores. This can be very common. We have recently reported our observations from Vancouver that about 20 percent of all prodromes will "abort" without further lesion development, even in the absence of any treatment.

While the prodromal is active, however, in order to be safest, herpes should be considered to be active for a short time. Examine yourself after the warning is over. Sometimes people who feel they do not get sores after the prodrome are not looking closely enough. Women with herpes must learn to use a mirror. Preferably the mirror will have a well-magnified side. Use a flashlight or some other light source that can be brought near to the skin. Remember that sores can vary and they may be very small. They may not hurt much. If no signs of herpes occur on the skin, wait a couple of days and resume normal skin contact. If sores develop, follow the phases and wait until the herpes is inactive. It may turn out that many of these "false prodromes" are just that—false. They may be only fleeting neuralgia from the last episode.

False prodromes also occur in some people taking oral acyclovir regularly for prevention of recurrences. It is as if the recurrent episode begins in the nerve and cycles on but is then aborted before the development of a visible lesion. The significance of these short episodes is unknown. For now, treat them as if they were short recurrences, whether they occur on acyclovir or off.

Can herpes cause headaches?

Yes, indeed, there is a herpes headache. Headache is a very common event during a true genital herpes primary infection. Primary herpes occasionally may be complicated by a syndrome called meningitis. The headache with meningitis is generally quite severe. It may be associated with other symptoms, such as stiff neck, nausea, and pain from bright light and loud noises. If this occurs during primary herpes, your doctor may choose to perform a lumbar puncture (needle in the low back) so that a sample of spinal fluid may be examined. This is a very safe procedure and generally causes about the same amount of discomfort as a blood test. Some people will, ironically, get a headache from the lumbar puncture test. The test will not be necessary in every case of primary herpes, only those where meningitis is considered significant. This is important in some cases to make sure that other causes for meningitis are not present. Herpes meningitis is generally benign; that is, it gets better on its own without treatment and generally does not recur.

Alternatively, headache may be the symptom of a prodromal. In other words, it may herald the onset of a new recurrence. Generally, this headache is mild and has no known cause. In fact, most headaches have no known cause. Being sick with anything can give a headache. Fever can bring on a headache. Tension from herpes or anything else can bring on a headache. If headaches are very severe, whether you feel they are related to herpes or not, you should discuss it with your doctor. Herpes should not generally be called a cause for chronic headache.

What other symptoms can herpes cause?

Genital herpes is still a poorly understood disease. We do not know how many people have it or how many know they have it. We do not know everything it can do. We do not know how often babies are affected. We do not know if it causes cancer. We probably only know some of the symptoms.

Once again, the symptoms of herpes are usually related to the sores. If they are near the urethra, it may hurt to urinate. If they are on the buttocks, it may hurt to sit. Sometimes, however, herpes causes invisible problems. Some people complain of recurring leg pain. This is usually in the back, radiating down the back of one leg. It may occur in the thigh. It is probably related to herpes. Occasionally, this pain may occur without any sores, like a false prodromal. If it is **episodic** (comes and goes) and is usually followed by sores on the skin, then it likely is a prodromal and should be considered a sign of active herpes. If the pain is **chronic** (always there or takes weeks to go away), chances are it will not be related to herpes. With chronic pain, other causes must be ruled out by a physician, and the presence of pain will have very little to do with virus activity on the skin. Persistent pain after herpes simplex or herpes zoster infection is over is called **postherpetic neuralgia.**

During primary infection any number of unusual things may occur. Primary herpes is an illness affecting the whole body. Meningitis, as previously described, is common during primary herpes. Other very rare severe consequences have resulted from herpes, including paralysis from a complication called **ascending myelitis.** This is so rare that only one or two cases in the world have ever been proven to be related to herpes. Temporary difficulties with urination or weakness in some muscles may occur more commonly. Even these are unusual, and if they should occur, function almost always fully reverts back to normal after a few weeks.

Occasionally a patient with herpes will get abdominal (stomach) pains from primary herpes. I have been told about patients who have actually undergone surgery for appendicitis, only to find out they have primary genital herpes. I should point out, however, that gonorrhea and Chlamydia are very common causes of a syndrome called **pelvic inflammatory disease (PID),** which often causes lower abdominal pain and may result in sterility. These are much more likely to cause abdominal pain than is herpes. In addition, they need to be treated by a trained person who must look for them and take a culture in order to identify them.

Erythema multiforme is a curious disease. It causes a skin rash which may look like rings of redness with central color changes (target lesions). A photograph of this problem is shown in Figure 13. In addition, the mucous membranes of the mouth, eyes (conjunctiva), or genitals may ulcerate and get painful and raw. As opposed to the ulcers of active herpes phases, these ulcers are not infectious. They are generally thought to be a hyperimmune reaction. In other words, the immune system of the body has not only responded, but it has "overresponded," resulting in cessation of the active virus infection. A few normal cells are damaged by the immune reaction as well, resulting in a rash and ulcers. One of the many causes of this unusual disease is herpes simplex. Any one individual with herpes is very unlikely to develop the problem. The treatment of this syndrome is sometimes simple and sometimes difficult. Cortisone may be called for here and it is usually taken by mouth rather than as a cream. The disease may relapse. It needs medical attention. Treatment with acyclovir is often advisable when this syndrome develops. Discuss treatment with your physician.

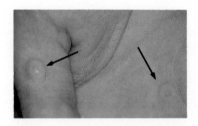

13. *A picture of the appearance of skin in a person with erythema multiforme. This is a "target" or "iris" lesion. The person has these sores, which come and go from time to time when he gets a fever blister. These sores are not infectious.*

Now that I have herpes, am I especially prone to other infections?

Herpes infection does not make you more susceptible to anything. Not long ago doctors were taught that secondary infection of the skin was a common complication of herpes, for example, a **staph** infection or **impetigo** from herpes. This is now known to be false. More than 99 percent of people with herpes have no other infection. Rarely, staph or strep (two common and easily treated bacteria) will invade the skin at the site broken by a herpes sore.

Because you have been affected by a sexually transmitted disease, there is a small statistical risk that you will have acquired another infection at the same time. This has nothing to do with your susceptibility but rather with your statistical chances of having "caught" something else. This means that the other infections commonly sexually transmitted (gonorrhea, Chlamydia, Trichomonas), and those easily confused with herpes by the way they look (syphilis, chancroid, shingles) should be ruled out. This is discussed in detail in Chapter 4.

Persons whose immunity is compromised from something unrelated, for example, patients with cancer, lymphoma, leukemia, transplantation, or acquired immune deficiency syndrome (AIDS) may occasionally get herpes simplex infections that do not heal readily. This occurs because of their immunity problem, not because of herpes. Herpes itself does not make these people susceptible. Rather, their immunity problems make them more susceptible to problematic herpes.

4

GENITAL HERPES: THE DIAGNOSIS

Choice is future oriented and never fully expressed in present action. It requires what is most distinctive about human reasoning: intention—the capacity to envisage and to compare future possibilities, to make estimates, sometimes to take indirect routes to a goal or to wait.

SISSELA BOK,
Secrets: On the Ethics of Concealment and Revelation

How is the diagnosis made?

In some situations, genital herpes may be a simple diagnosis for the general practitioner. It may elude the specialist in others. When symptoms and signs of herpes are "classical," that is, when a known exposure has taken place and sores have developed that are painful clustered vesicles (blisters) or ulcers on a red, inflamed base, the clinical diagnosis is clear-cut. Recurrences make herpes even more likely. Then, the virus itself is detected by a culture test from one of the sores, confirming the diagnosis. In order to make sure that no other diseases accompany the herpes, tests for syphilis, gonorrhea, Chlamydia, trichomonas and yeast are also performed.

On the other hand, certain people with genital herpes have mild intermittent symptoms. The only sore might be a pinpoint, single ulcer on the labia that lasts for a few days and comes every six months. It may not hurt at all. The diagnosis may not occur to the patient or the physician, leading only to confusion. If the possibility is considered, a virus culture test to detect herpes in the sore should be obtained during an active phase of infection. If the test is positive, herpes is likely to be the cause of the sore.

If the test is negative, however, herpes may or may not be the cause of the problem. Remember the discussion about the phases of herpes (Chapter 3). Was the test obtained during an active period? If not, it can be expected to be negative, even if herpes is the problem. Even if the period was an active one, quite often herpes virus is not recoverable. How was the test obtained? Was the doctor's office far away from the laboratory? If so, the virus may not have survived the trip. How experienced is the laboratory? This may vary. Even under ideal circumstances, virus recovery in the laboratory after only one try is not always possible.

If you suspect herpes and your doctor agrees, your best bet is to return again for virus culture at the *first* sign of recurrence. The earlier the specimen is obtained, the better is the chance of an accurate test. In my experience, two visits will suffice, *if* the visits are early. If we suspect herpes very strongly, however, we will keep culturing until we find it. Rarely, four or five tests are necessary.

I have been exposed to herpes. Should I go to my doctor now for a test?

This is an increasingly more common story. It is also a difficult problem. If you have been exposed to someone with herpes, the person may have been in an active stage or an inactive stage.

If the lesion was in an inactive stage, your risk is very low. If no symptoms develop, do nothing and try to relax. Nothing will almost certainly be what continues to happen unless you become exposed, in the future, to an active infection.

If the infection was in an active stage, you may have been exposed. Whether you will develop herpes or not will depend upon several factors.

Was there virus present? The active stages are a good guess for when exposure risk is high, but often a sore may have no living virus in it. If sores were active, you may have been infected, but not necessarily so.

The inoculum is probably important. If the number of virus particles (inoculum) that have made contact was very high, then infection is more likely. If virus is present in very small amounts, infection is less likely.

Where did inoculation take place? Was this contact through thin skin, for instance, on the genitals? Were there cuts on the skin? Was contact prolonged? Did a long time elapse before washing the area? All of these things might increase the chance for any virus to transfer from one person to another.

Several other "host factors" also play a role. If you have antibody to herpes, a higher "dose" may be required to result in illness. The immune system may also be an important factor in some ways we do not understand.

What really matters, however, is whether or not you develop symptoms of herpes, assuming you know what they are. If no symptoms are present, a trip to the doctor will not assure you that you do not have herpes. A doctor can only tell you if herpes sores are seen at the time you are examined, on the areas examined. If symptoms develop, e.g., vaginal discharge, sores, unexplained tenderness of the genitals, redness, pimples or swollen lymph nodes, then go to the doctor *without delay*. If no other obvious cause for the symptoms is present and your exposure to herpes is likely, inform the doctor and ask for a herpes culture. Remember, go early when the symptoms are present. Waiting it out does not help. Herpes will go away on its own temporarily, only to possibly return again. If you want to know (and it is your responsibility to know), go to the doctor when symptoms first appear.

If you feel your exposure to an active herpes sore was fairly certain and if this happened within the last few days, you might consider the possibility of taking a course of oral acyclovir *before* developing symptoms (see Chapter 11).

How is the diagnosis proven?

The only way to prove that herpes is present, regardless of

how sure it looks, is with a test that shows herpes simplex virus to be present in a sore. The most sensitive test (the most likely to show positive when it is herpes) is a culture test. Since virus lives inside cells, a few of those cells from a sore must be taken and sent for culture. This is easy to do by just rolling a wet cotton or dacron swab into a sore. The swab is then placed into a special salt solution and sent to the laboratory.

At the lab, some of the fluid is removed and placed onto healthy human cells that are kept growing in tubes. The cells are called a tissue culture. Once virus is placed onto the cells, this is called a virus culture. The laboratory technologist will then keep the cells growing at body temperature in an incubator. During the next several days, the technician removes the culture from the incubator and places the tube under the microscope. If the cells remain healthy, then the culture is negative. If the cells become sick from herpes, they will round up and group themselves together. This change in appearance is called the **cytopathic effect (CPE).** An area of herpes infection of cells called **fibroblasts** is shown in Figure 14. Note the long, pointed, wispy appearance of the normal cells on the right. Compare this to the sick-appearing, swollen cells where the virus is growing (to the left of the bracket).

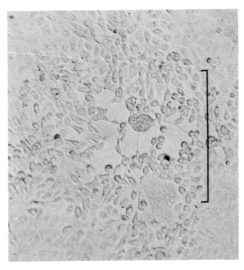

14. Microscopic appearance of cells affected by herpes simplex virus. Normal cells in culture are altered by the infection taking place in the test tube. Cells are swollen and fused. This is called cytopathic effect (or CPE) and is suggestive of herpes simplex infection.

Once the CPE has occurred, a small number of cells are removed from the tube and placed onto a slide. The technician will then add a herpes simplex antibody to the slide. This antibody is usually attached to a chemical which will **fluoresce** (emit light) under ultraviolet (UV) light. If the cells fluoresce, the changes in the cells must be certainly caused by herpes simplex: the positive culture test. A positive fluorescence test is shown in Figure 15. The bright areas on the cells are fluorescing because herpes antibody is stuck to the virus on the cell.

15. *Infected cells under the microscope are flooded with a herpes antibody attached to a fluorescent dye. Infected areas "shine" under the ultraviolet light.*

Several other methods of diagnosis may also be used. If fluid is present, e.g., inside a vesicle, the virus may be seen under the electron microscope. This is a very powerful (and very expensive) microscope about the size of a small car. An experienced and capable technician must operate the machine. Identification of "herpes-like particles" is truly an art. Interpretation may be very difficult and, unfortunately, occasionally misleading. Remember, all herpes viruses look the same under the electron microscope. Nobody can say if the virus is Type 1 or Type 2 or even if it is shingles just from this test. Furthermore, even though the machine is powerful, it is not sensitive. One must have a lot of virus in a very carefully collected specimen in order to obtain a positive electron microscope test. One must further have great faith in the talents of the technician. A picture of herpes simplex virus in the electron microscope is seen in Figure 16.

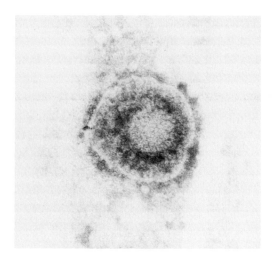

16. *An electron microscope takes a picture of herpes directly. The regular microscope cannot see with such intense magnification. The electron microscope shows the enveloped virus. Within the envelope, the nucleocapsid containing 162 capsomeres, shaped like an icosahedron, can be detected if your imagination is good.*

The fluorescent antibody technique described above for cells in culture may also be attempted directly on clinical specimens. A smear from the sore can also be placed onto a microscope slide and examined directly (a Pap smear). Since herpes may result in the formation of giant cells, these may be seen in the microscope directly. Special stains can be done on the slide and then it is called a **Tzanck smear.**

These smears and the fluorescence and electron microscopy tests and others being developed are quick tests. In general, compared to culture tests, quick answer tests sacrifice a bit of accuracy for speed or convenience. Which test to do depends on the situation. Sometimes it may be necessary to do more than one type of test.

Each of these methods provides direct evidence of herpes infection and, if positive, proves that herpes is present. Remember, if one specific virus test should be negative, this does not prove that herpes was not present. If there is a negative finding, it is always much more difficult (and sometimes impossible) to prove that herpes is *not* causing a genital sore.

Is there a blood test for herpes?

Can I take a blood test to determine the presence of herpes virus? Yes. Is it helpful? Not generally. Can the result be interpreted to tell you if you have herpes? Not usually. What is the test? It is a test to measure herpes antibody and to say how much herpes antibody is present in the blood. This it will do, but the vast majority of herpes antibody tests are not type-specific. That is, they cannot usually tell the difference, with absolute accuracy, between past infection with Type 1 or Type 2. Antibody of some type may be present in 50 to 80 percent of people by the age of 20. So what will a positive test tell you about herpes? Really very little. Sometimes people look for a rising amount of antibody to herpes from one time to another—termed acute and convalescent. Unfortunately, this is usually inaccurate also. Conversely, some people with culture-proven genital herpes have negative antibody tests. Forget about herpes blood tests except in very unusual circumstances. A single blood test will not tell you with certainty if you have genital herpes. If two tests were done, however, and the first was completely negative and the second was definitely positive, and if your infection was your very first, this pattern would be suggestive. Someday, possibly soon, a blood test will become available that is reliably type-specific. These tests are not generally available yet. In the proper setting, an antibody test may offer useful extra information. For now, a blood test cannot diagnose if herpes is present or not.

What type of doctor should I go to?

If you have a good relationship with your family doctor you may wish to start there. Ask the questions you need to ask. Find out whether your symptoms are suggestive of herpes. If you need more detailed answers to your questions, you may ask to be sent to a clinic for sexually transmitted diseases or to a specialist in the area. Your physician should be able to guide you to a gynecologist, dermatologist, urologist, specialist in infectious diseases, or someone who has some special experience with herpes. It matters little how much or what type of special training the physician or health practitioner has. It is information and accuracy that you need. You must work with your health practitioner. He or she is the only person who can use the proper tests to help you find out if you have herpes. Only a trained professional can arrange for the other tests you will need to be sure you have nothing else that requires specific treatment.

Does it matter if the herpes is Type 1 or Type 2?

As a general rule, herpes simplex is herpes simplex. Type 1 may cause genital herpes. In general, however, in North America, 80 to 90 percent of genital herpes is caused by Type 2. Some infections are caused by mixtures of both types. Scientists have observed that Type 1 genital herpes recurs much less often than Type 2. The reason for this is unknown. More than 95 percent of persons with *recurrent* herpes will be having a Type 2 recurrence. By contrast, a *primary* genital infection from a Type 1 infection is very common.

Therapy is now available for treatment of herpes infections. Some (not all) therapy which is being developed is type-specific. If type-specific therapy becomes a clinical reality, then typing will become an obvious necessity. Some laboratories now do herpes typing routinely. In the recent past, typing was a difficult thing to do well, but the laboratory methods for proper typing are now much easier, and they will become easier yet in the very near future.

During the very first episode of genital herpes it is a good idea to insist that the virus be typed accurately, since Type 1 and Type 2 have very different prognoses. In other words, most Type 1 primary outbreaks recur only rarely, and some, not at all. Thus, it is reassuring to find out during this primary episode which type you have, should it turn out to be Type 1. Since recurrent herpes has already established its pattern, typing is of little clinical consequence in this setting.

Ways have now been devised for "fingerprinting" the virus. As a special research tool, it is possible to tell one person's virus from another by its "DNA fingerprint." This method has allowed us to trace outbreaks of infection to the source. It seems that the number of possible differences, in this virus, from strain to strain, are nearly infinite. These tools remain in the hands of the researchers for now, although determination of whether your virus is Type 1 or Type 2 herpes has now become routinely available.

5

GENITAL HERPES: TRANSMISSION

*Any disease that is treated as a mystery and acutely enough feared
will be felt to be morally if not literally contagious.*
SUSAN SONTAG,
Illness as Metaphor

How does herpes spread from person to person?

In order to infect a new host, the herpes virus must attach to
the epithelial (skin) cells of the body. It must use its envelope,
which helps it to hook onto the new cell. The virus will live
only a very short time outside of a cell. Without its surrounding
envelope, the virus dries out and is rendered "sterile." Furthermore, anything which might dissolve the envelope, like
soap or alcohol, will effectively neutralize the virus. It cannot
be sent across the open spaces (in a room by sneezing, for example), for it dries out quickly.

Probably, a certain required number of virus particles must
reach epithelial cells in the new host for infection to be successful. Using large numbers is nature's way of compensating
for the failure of most particles to set up effectively in their
new host. For example, even though pregnancy results from
the union of only one sperm and one egg, millions of sperm are
required to ensure that one gets through to its target. How
many herpes virus particles are needed for transmission? This
is now unknown and will probably remain unknown, since the

human experiment required to find the answer is not an ethical one to perform. One can easily imagine, however, that if a very small number of particles were to infect a cell, the reproduction process of the virus might lag behind the immunological defense network within the host working to halt the process. That network is much like an army with specialized units. These units have a certain starting force and reinforcements are always on the way, capable of building up each battalion. If the invasion force (the virus) is very small, no reinforcements are needed and the invasion is quashed. If the invasion force is strong, there is a delay until reinforcements come. During the delay, disease occurs. Because of this numbers game, combined with the fact that virus dies upon drying, direct inoculation is generally required for herpes to spread.

This direct inoculation occurs when infected epithelial cells from one person, preferably kept moist and warm at body temperature, helped by rubbing and, even better, by scratching, come in direct contact with the epithelial cells of another person. Regular skin, like on the hand, is protected against all but the most massive invasion because of a natural barrier on the skin called keratin. Keratin is waxy and strong. Just as it repels water, it repels herpes virus particles (see Figure 1). Unless the keratin is torn, in a cut for instance, the virus does not make it to an epithelial cell. In mucous membranes, however, like those lining the mouth, eye, and genital area, the barrier is very thin. The epithelial cells are waiting, exposed, very near the skin surface. This is where herpes tends to take up initial residence, for this is where access is easiest. It does not take much imagination, then, to see how herpes gets where it is going. On one person, an active lesion with herpes growing and alive; add friction for heat and for removal of infected cells from the surface of the donor; add moisture for easy travel and to prevent drying; add exposed epithelial cells of another person, and a new infection is the result.

Thus, genital herpes tends to be sexually transmitted. Other types of transmission are possible, but not usual. One can imagine that most contact between two persons involving the genitals is going to be sexually oriented. This type of sexual transmission does not require penetration (penis into vagina). It could be mouth to vagina; mouth to penis; penis to mouth; finger to penis; penis to anus—or any other combination. The requirements are only infected cells and exposure to new cells along with heat and moisture. Herpes does not care if there is sex happening. Sure, herpes likes sex, but it also likes kissing and wrestling and rugby, and any other "contact sport" that gives it the new environmental opportunities it constantly seeks.

What can be done to prevent herpes from spreading?

For herpes to move from one person to another it must be active—*growing*—on the skin or mucous membrane. It does not jump from its latent site in the ganglion to the genitals of another. When skin herpes is active, protection is achieved by completely *avoiding* sore-to-skin contact. A condom or foam or avoiding vaginal penetration does not offer sufficient protection when a sore is present.

Anywhere herpes is *active* is a place to avoid having contact. If it is in the mouth, then avoid kissing, oral sex, and so on. If on the finger, keep your hand to yourself while your infection is active. If it is on your thigh, watch what rubs against your partner (try bandaging it). If it is on the genitals, *avoid genital contact*.

You need not avoid kissing with active herpes unless sores are on your mouth, just as people with cold sores on the mouth needn't avoid genital contact—just kissing. In other words, active herpes is a time to avoid contact with affected areas, but *not a time to avoid contact altogether*. It is a time for creative contact. You have probably always had sexual contact during which you carefully avoided putting your finger into your partner's eye. This has never concerned you. Now, in somewhat the same way, you must learn to have contact while avoiding the area of skin *actively* affected with herpes. This is critical. Total abstinence is okay for a while, but it leads to changes in self-image which are not necessary or useful. They will be discussed later.

You think your active phases are over, but you're worried, you're not sure. Then you might want to consider using condoms along with the spermicidal agent, **nonoxynol-9.** More information on the use of condoms and safer sex techniques is available in Chapter 12. However, during the inactive phases of infection, condoms may reduce the small risk of transmission even further and enhance your peace of mind. If your symptoms are over, chances are you've got no virus left on the skin. If you do, chances are it is a small amount. Should this event arise while you are using condoms properly (see Chapter 12), the chances of avoiding transmission are strongly in your favor. Some people (not all) find that in the beginning—for the first several months after their initial herpes—that this business of telling one phase from the next is tricky. With careful attention to your body during this period, an awareness generally comes quite easily. One gets to know one's herpes. During this getting-to-know-period, condoms are strongly recommended.

Could I spread the herpes from the genitals to my eyes? My fingers? My mouth? My brain?

This question is an extremely common and important one. The name for spreading infection from one part of your body to another is "autoinoculation." If one area on your body can be affected, why not everywhere? Can herpes move around?

The answer first requires some background information. If you broke a herpes vesicle (blister) during the active period with a needle and stuck this needle into your arm or your eye or your lip or even your brain, for that matter, you would probably develop a new infection in that new site. Injection into the arm was actually tried on volunteers several years ago. Recently I saw an individual who thought that breaking herpes blisters with a needle might help them to heal. Unfortunately he once accidentally stuck his finger with the needle after breaking his blisters and now has herpes recurring on his finger. Aside from such extreme circumstances, however, herpes very rarely gets into the blood or any other part of the person affected except for the **skin** and the local **sensory nerves** in the area. It does not get tossed around from organ to organ. For the most part, it stays where it is. Reasonable personal hygiene is a good rule. Since genital herpes is generally held within the confines of underwear, the problem is minimal.

Another person I've seen gets recurrent cold sores. He gets his herpes outbreaks twice a year—usually on the corner of his nose. One August, during an active outbreak, the pollen was heavy in the air. His hay fever was in full bloom along with the flowers. He sneezed and he sneezed. He rubbed his itchy eyes and he rubbed some more. Later he noticed the appearance of herpes sores on his eyelids. While this is an example of Type 1 autoinoculation, the general principles are the same as for Type 2. Extreme circumstances can, rarely, result in autoinoculation.

Often the question is asked, could you give yourself genital herpes by rubbing a sore on your mouth and then touching your own genitals. This type of infection has never been documented and for several reasons is extremely unlikely to occur. First, the dose required for autoinoculation is probably very high. The people in the examples above were able to do this only under unusual and extreme circumstances (needles, and hayfever with cold sores).

During primary genital herpes, you could more easily autoinoculate. For example, vaginal secretions naturally ooze down over the perineum, where new sores may develop before your body has developed strong immunity to herpes, which takes a couple of weeks after the first infection starts. Remember the rule with herpes—there is no jumping from place to place. But put enough virus *directly* into a new place and new infection may occur. Autoinoculation is much more likely to occur during the initial attack, especially if it is a true primary. At that time, the immune defenses like antibodies and lymphocytes are not yet operating at full steam, and therefore little obstruction lies in the path of virus, anxious to move on to new places. Immunity will largely prevent this spreading, so once the primary episode is over, the amount of virus required for new sores to take root will be much higher. Immunity alone, however, is not enough of a defense against a lot of virus.

Stick to good hygiene. Think about what you are doing when you touch your sores. Wash your hands afterwards. Keep contact lenses out of your mouth the same way you should keep them away from your genitals. If sores are active, don't wipe your genitals and then rub your face with the same cloth. However, transmission to your eyes from your own genitals is talked about often, but seen almost never. Of 2,000 patients I have personally seen with genital herpes, only one has had an eye infection. It may have been inoculated there at the same time it was inoculated onto the genitals. Autoinoculation in that situation is unlikely. As you can see, genital herpes is not a blinding disease.

Genital herpes can affect the nervous system. It is not associated with herpes encephalitis in adults. Sometimes it causes an inflammation of the protective sac around the brain called the meninges. The inflammation is called aseptic meningitis. It will not damage the brain or you. It may cause a severe headache (see Chapter 3). Encephalitis, or brain infection, is no more (or less) likely to happen to the person with genital herpes than it is to anyone else. It is rare, confusing, difficult, and dangerous, but not associated with genital herpes at all. Nongenital herpes infections are extensively discussed in Chapter 10.

Could I spread herpes without sexual intercourse, e.g., to my children?

At the risk of sounding repetitive, *direct* contact is required in order to contract herpes—not sexual contact. If your child's skin touches your herpes, then yes, of course it can spread. In fact, most herpes begins in childhood when the baby or child is kissed by a relative or friend with active Type 1 herpes on his or her mouth.

Objects which pass quickly from one person to another are, theoretically, a possible source as well. For example, if you share a drinking cup or a cigarette while you have a cold sore, transmission is possible. How about a bath towel? I would suggest not using the same towel with others while lesions are active. That would logically go for underwear and other intimate articles. Simple washing of towels or other articles is sufficient to dissolve the herpes envelope and will kill the virus effectively. There is no need to use special disinfectants or virus killers. Plain soap is perfect. In fact, there is no good evidence that sharing of bath articles has ever caused one case of herpes, but why risk it? Not sharing underwear seems like a small price to pay! Despite lots of headlines about towels, toilet seats, articles in doctors' offices, and even hot tubs and water slides, no evidence for transmission in these ways has been found. The best evidence is that children are not flocking to physicians with genital herpes. Patients with genital herpes generally avoid giving genital herpes to their children because they do not have sexual contact with their children. It's that simple. That is not to imply that rare exceptions don't exist, because they probably do. You need do no more for prevention, however, than use reasonable personal hygiene.

What about toilet seats?

The toilet seat argument has been around since toilet seats were invented. Researchers have looked for gonorrhea, syphilis, you name it, on toilet seats. Herpes that gets onto a toilet seat, especially a wet warm one that has not been cleaned in a few days, can stay alive there for a while. It does not stay very healthy. It begins to die as soon as it leaves the skin, but it takes a while. If dried or cleaned it disappears. If it stays wet it may take an hour or two to fizzle. Even if herpes were alive on the seat, transmission to the next person by this method would be unlikely. The back of the thigh and the buttocks are thick-skinned areas, relatively resistant to penetration by virus. The temperature and moisture settings are wrong for transmission. In fact, no cases of herpes from toilet seats or from any other inanimate objects (swimming pools, saunas, water slides) have ever been proven. Experiments suggesting toilet seats as a source for herpes have never provided any evidence whatsoever for transmission. Rather, they have concluded that toilet seats that are not disinfected do not actively kill the virus. Instead, the virus dies slowly on its own.

However, I have spent a lot of time on toilet seats in my life and have often wondered how a sexually transmissible virus could get onto the seat in the first place. Certainly if sores are present at the bottom of the buttocks, or if they reside on the back of the thigh, then they touch the seat. I do recommend that people with sores in those places use toilet paper or seat covers while the sores are in their active phases. They might consider drying off the seat for others, or using a pocket-sized wet napkin. If your sores are on the penis, the labia, the pubic area or the mouth, the problem is avoided by keeping those areas away from contact with the seat. Now this seems straightforward to me. The overwhelming majority of people with herpes never contact the seat with their sores unless they have unusual personal habits. An elder colleague of mine, upon reading about the toilet seat issue in the newspaper, suggested that herpes is transmitted in public toilets only when two people make love in the stall!

No, there should not be separate toilets for people with herpes. Yes, my personal bias and infectious disease background would suggest that daily disinfection of toilets is a good idea and that toilet seat covers are not a bad commodity. However, these suggestions will help to prevent infectious hepatitis and typhoid fever much more than syphilis or herpes. For herpes, the toilet seat issue is almost an academic one.

Can I spread herpes without having sores?

Not having sores means different things to different people. If a person has herpes enough times to recognize the phases, if these phases are very clearly understood, if healing is clearly recognized, then the risk of transmission is very small. Remember, herpes cannot jump from the latent ganglion site to the genitals of another. Occasionally, in some people, active herpes is totally asymptomatic (without symptoms) even after it has been symptomatic (with symptoms). For the most part, however, what seems to be asymptomatic really means that certain symptoms have not been recognized as herpes. In other words, the hemorrhoid that suddenly swells up and itches is usually just a hemorrhoid. Occasionally, however, it is herpes. That intermittent pain in the leg could be a herpes prodromal. The itch in the pubic hair is probably a pimple or just an itch. It could be herpes. The sore throat you have may be a cold. It may be herpes. The list is endless. This all really means the same old thing; get to know your herpes. If you are aware of where it might be likely to bother you, avoid contact when an unusual symptom arises. Wait and see. Do blisters or ulcers (even very small ones) ever develop? If not, your itch is probably just an itch.

This risk of spreading herpes when you do not have any symptoms is small—very small. In a recent study by Dr. Vontver and his coworkers in Seattle, the risk of having a no-symptoms, no-sores, culture-positive recurrence was studied in pregnant women. In the absence of visible lesions, herpes was isolated in 7 of 1,068 (0.66 percent) cervical cultures and 8 of 1,068 (0.75 percent) external genital cultures. Another study of a similar nature (in pregnancy) performed by Dr. J.H. Harger and coworkers in Pittsburgh suggested an asymptomatic rate of virus shedding of about 3 percent. Numbers will depend upon the persons undergoing study (how well they know their herpes), the sensitivity of the laboratory (how much virus is necessary to get a positive test), and the care of the physician responsible for looking for sores (is this really asymptomatic or missed symptomatic?). The risk of transmission during inactive phases is small. Another study in 26 patients with frequent genital herpes was reported by Dr. Straus and his associates from the National Institutes of Health. He cultured these volunteers every day! Asymptomatic shedding over 11 months occurred in 8 per 1,000 cultures. This accounted for 28 asymptomatic episodes in 26 people, each asymptomatic episode lasting an average of 1.54 days. So, it happens—just not very often or for very long.

In fact, people with herpes may be better equipped to reduce the risk of transmission by avoiding sore contact during active phases of infection than are people who think they do not have herpes. People who think they do not have herpes at all do not know what an itch may be and may never consider the active phases of herpes in themselves. This disease is so common that sexual contact with anyone in the 1980s is going to be a significant risk for herpes. The risk within the herpes group is no greater than the rest, depending upon the people involved. It just requires care and learning about yourself. The person with herpes who is educated about the active phases of infection may, in some ways, be at an advantage since there is a clear course of action for avoiding transmission. On the other hand, the person who thinks he or she has no herpes (and is mistaken) will be a likely source of infection. The careful, informed individual who has symptomatic herpes can do a great deal to prevent spreading the infection.

If I have herpes, am I immune to a second infection from someone else?

No. In 1980, a study done in Atlanta, Georgia, offered proof that genital herpes can recur with more than one strain of the virus, suggesting that patients with one herpes can get another. Since immunity is important, it is generally thought that getting your second herpes is a little more difficult than the first. The antibody makes it more difficult and protects somewhat, but sex during active herpes can give a second infection.

It is a painstaking effort to tell one herpes strain from another, but it can be done. This test is not something your family doctor can perform. In order to tell the herpes of Mr. Jones from the herpes of Ms. Smith, a "DNA fingerprint" is performed. The virus is grown in large amounts in the laboratory and is purified and the DNA (see Chapter 1) is extracted with chemicals. Then special enzymes called restriction endonucleases are added, which cut the DNA in several special places. These small pieces that are left are then placed into a "gel," which is much like unflavoured gelatin—wobbly, but firm. An electric charge is added and the pieces travel inside the gel. Since small pieces travel faster than large ones, the gel makes a "fingerprint." Then, subtle differences between one virus strain and another can be detected. Using this method, several investigators have shown differences in the fingerprints between virus strains. Dual infections occurring with two strains at the same time, or two strains on separate recurrences in the same individual, have been demonstrated.

Despite this, second infections with a new strain are considered, for practical purposes, to be an extremely unusual, if not rare, occurrence.

How could this happen to me?

Herpes infection can happen to anyone. Several studies have proven this. Not too many years ago, you were considered to be at greater risk of acquiring herpes if you were poor. More recently, the Herpes Resource Center, an organization devoted to helping people with herpes, reported a study of over 3,000 affected persons. They found that people with herpes (in their organization) often came from a high socioeconomic level (56 percent earned over $20,000 per year in 1981) and were highly educated (53 percent completed four years of college). Even this study does not represent the average person with herpes. It is not money or education or class that will determine if you get herpes. Even sexual habits may or may not correlate in any one individual to the acquisition of this infection. Obviously, since herpes is almost always sexually transmitted, some type of sexual contact is usual. By statistical chances alone, anyone with more sexual contacts is more likely to acquire this virus. However, herpes has become so universal that often there is a history of just one or two sexual contacts in a lifetime. Since this is usually an external disease, that sexual contact does not have to include vaginal penetration. Several well-documented cases of herpes in women who are virgins have been described, almost always the result of an oral-to-genital encounter.

As a society, we have subjected ourselves to a higher chance of running into herpes partially by giving up condoms and foam for the convenience of the intrauterine device (IUD) and the pill. We run into herpes more often because sex has become less and less forbidden over the last few years. Oral-to-genital sex has also become commonplace, making the likelihood of oral-to-genital transmission of herpes more likely. Sexual transmission is only required as the last event in genital herpes. Since herpes infection of some type is found in most people on this earth, we are talking about obtaining an infection that is almost more normal to have than to not have. When sores occur on the genitals, however, the emotional impact is greater than the same infection on the mouth. Realize that this stigma is mainly a media phenomenon and not an affliction unique to you. You have a nuisance skin affliction which comes and goes. It has unusual complications that are unlikely to occur and are highly preventable.

It has been suggested by some that the growth of herpes is a new demonstration of the "wrath of God." In response to this, I would point out that elimination of all but monogamous sexual contact would cut down the overall incidence of this infection, but monogamy would not eliminate herpes. A monogamous individual, and even a sexually inactive individual, could get genital herpes. It is, in fact, scientifically accurate to state that increasing the numbers of sexual partners statistically increases the chances of getting any sexually transmitted disease. From the prevention point of view, it is, and always was, wise to be selective, to know your partner, to avoid casual sex, etc. Religious preference does not correlate in any way to susceptibility to infection, however. Herpes is no more a sign of punishment from God than Legionnaire's disease was a sign of punishment from God inflicted upon the American Legion. Ascribing any new disease or affliction, or any old disease or affliction, to the plagues of God is rewriting the Bible. In the case of herpes, it is also the the result of misinformation.

I had sex last night and awoke with a sore.
Did I spread it to my partner?

Probably not, if you had no symptoms of active infection when you had genital contact. Awakening with a sore seems to happen frequently to people with herpes. It is probably not significant. Such a circumstance obviously depends upon the frequency with which you have sex. If sexual contact is a daily occurrence, then *every time* you awake with herpes you will have had sex the night before. Herpes shedding does not generally begin before the symptoms of an outbreak. If you have followed the guidelines for preventing transmission, you should not fear. If you think that exposure to herpes did occur (e.g., you are not sure about when your symptoms began), then your partner may wish to consider using oral acyclovir in this circumstance (see Chapter 11).

Can I have a long-term relationship with one person and never transmit herpes?

Yes, such relationships are very common. In general, the chances of missing an active sore have got to be higher as the number of encounters between any two people increase. It is often the case, however, that the couple who transmit herpes after several years together with only one partner affected remember an event during which the barrier to active infection broke down. Scientists admit that transmission can occasionally occur in the absence of sores, so it would be misleading to say that transmission is 100 percent preventable. Nothing in biology is 100 percent certain.

Furthermore, in time, some couples lose their desire to hold to strict rules in avoiding transmission. Since herpes is usually physically mild, some people in permanent relationships may decide the prevention is not worthwhile. Risk taking may increase in frequency.

Speaking of risks, we take them all the time. We risk our lives driving in cars; we risk our genital health having sex. To take risks is human. To take risks with someone with herpes is also human, and, relative to other risks, not such a big risk. But choosing which risks are right for you is an individual choice. These types of choices must be left up to the individual and to the individual couple. A break in the barrier to active infection can occur because of mistake or because of choice, or less commonly, because of asymptomatic virus shedding.

6

HERPES OF THE NEWBORN

Every mother entertains the idea that her child will be a hero, thus showing her wonderment at the thought of engendering a being with consciousness and freedom; but she is also in dread of giving birth to a defective or a monster, because she is aware to what a frightening extent the welfare of the flesh is contingent upon circumstances —and this embryo dwelling within her is only flesh.

SIMONE DE BEAUVOIR,
The Second Sex

What is herpes of the newborn?

Despite dramatic breakthroughs in knowledge, our understanding of immunology (the defense network of the body) leaves a lot unexplained. The immunology of the newborn baby is especially confusing. At birth, an overwhelming number of changes take place in the infant. The heart begins pumping blood in a different direction, the lungs inflate with air for the first time, and the baby becomes a free-living organism facing the external environment. For reasons that are only partially understood, most babies thrive in this new environment. Others are highly susceptible to infection.

Many different infectious agents can cause infections in newborns under the right circumstances. Most of these agents would be entirely tolerable to an adult. They may even be "normal flora"—a part of the normal (indeed, necessary) colony of bacteria or fungi that cause absolutely no disease in the adult who harbors the organism. One example of normal flora would be a bacteria called **Escherichia coli.** These bacteria inhabit the gut of nearly everyone. Commonly, a woman will get some of these bacteria into her bladder—often the consequence of minor trauma from sexual contact—and a urinary tract infection (cystitis) will result.

Most babies also tolerate this organism. Essentially all babies are exposed to this organism during birth. Of 1,000 babies who are exposed, 998 could not care less. However, an unfortunate one or two of the thousand will develop severe, overwhelming infection—even meningitis—with this bacteria. These infants may suffer severe damage or even die from this infection with a "normal" agent. In some of these babies the reason for infection is obvious, for example, prolonged rupture of the membranes, where exposure of baby to bacteria may be very intense and sustained over a long period. In other cases the reasons for infection remain unknown.

Why should a newborn baby be so susceptible to infection? The possibilities are numerous. In every baby the immune system is somewhat immature. Immune experience is nearly as undeveloped as the baby's job experience at birth, except that the mother can give some immune experience to the baby by passing along some antibodies which filter across the placenta from the mother's blood. In this way newborns are born possessing many of the same antibodies as the mother—antibodies which are passed on from the mother to the fetus.

While inside the uterus, the fetus is essentially protected from most infection by the filtering capabilities of the placenta, which effectively exclude almost all infecting agents. This means that at the time of birth the newborn has never before had to respond with immunity to infection. All those lymphocytes and macrophages and so forth, which do the majority of immune fighting against foreign invaders, have never been stimulated before. Just as the newborn has never before seen the light of day, so his or her white blood cells have never seen a bacterium. The cells are just beginning to learn how the system works. Thus, occasionally, a baby will succumb to an infection which would cause a mild illness or no problem at all in you or me.

Herpes of the newborn is one example of this problem.

Herpes simplex, which causes a mild skin infection in the adult, may, under the right circumstances, overcome the immature immune system of a newborn baby and lead to overwhelming infection, which can disseminate throughout the body, result in encephalitis (brain infection) with consequent brain damage, or result in eye infection and eye damage. This type of problem is very unlikely to occur in any individual newborn. It is even unlikely to occur in any one individual born to a mother with genital herpes. Curiously, more than half of the babies born with this disease come from mothers who have never known they have herpes. In fact, once the mother knows she has genital herpes, newborn herpes becomes preventable. It needs to be considered so that the pregnancy can be properly watched. Herpes is not a reason to avoid having children, however, since the baby of a mother with genital herpes is unlikely to have any problems with neonatal (newborn) infection.

What are the signs?

Just as the symptoms of genital herpes vary, depending on the location of the infection, so do the signs of neonatal herpes vary with the location. In unusual cases, herpes may already be present at birth. Since infection usually begins at the time of birth, however, it most commonly takes several days to a couple of weeks to become evident. The most common herpes infection in newborns is probably on the skin. The skin sore looks much like that on an adult, i.e., a single vesicle (blister) or cluster of vesicles. Occasionally herpes may begin as a red rash or a purplish rash. Because many very mild skin rashes of infancy can mimic herpes, it is important to obtain a medical opinion when a skin rash develops in a newborn—especially if a sore develops which is similar to those pictured in Chapter 3. It is also important to remember that almost every baby has some type of skin rash at some point in the first few weeks of life. Normal things called milia, for example, which look like little pimples, may be frightening to the mother with genital herpes who thinks her baby has the infection. These are very, very common. Several babies in every nursery will have milia.

Expect to see a skin rash in your baby just because it is a baby. Talk it over with your doctor. Genuine herpes sores may be found anywhere on the skin, but especially on the head of a baby delivered the usual way (head first), the buttocks of a baby delivered by breech (rear first), and so on. The mouth is a common site also, as is anywhere in the scalp where a fetal scalp monitor might have been placed.

Another common site of involvement with herpes of the newborn is the eyes. Again, most babies have red and swollen eyes unrelated to herpes because of the silver nitrate placed there at birth to prevent infection. Generally, this redness and discharge fades quickly over the first few days of life. Herpes in the eye most often appears as redness—**conjunctivitis**—with or without discharge of pus from the eye. Herpes infection of the eye is often detectable only by special examinations done by an eye specialist (ophthalmologist).

The more severe neonatal herpes syndromes are infection of the central nervous system (the brain) and infection that disseminates (virus infection which is blood-borne and thus distributed in many parts of the body). Brain infection tends to appear late (from one to four weeks of age). An affected baby may suddenly lose his or her early very active behavior and become lethargic. The baby might stop caring about such things as feeding—or might do just the opposite, becoming very irritable. This, of course, is a very common thing in normal babies as well, but an irritable baby should be assessed to make *sure* it is "just colic." Shaking or twitching or fits (like epileptic fits) in an infant should be checked out by a physician without delay. Babies with herpes infection of the nervous system may have skin sores, but very often a baby with serious herpes infection will show no skin problem whatsoever.

The same is true for dissemination; that is, skin sores may be present, but lack of skin sores is also very common. This syndrome appears a bit earlier, often within the first seven days of life. Rarely, herpes may be present at birth, implying that herpes infected the baby inside the womb. There is no known specific method for prevention of womb infection. Most babies with dissemination have nonspecific symptoms, including lethargy, going off feeding, and vomiting. An affected baby may become gravely ill very rapidly. **Jaundice** (yellow skin) is a very common thing in infants. When associated with actual liver enlargement and abnormal blood tests of liver function, jaundice may be the result of herpes or it may be caused by many other things. Sometimes the infant with herpes gets **pneumonia,** has difficulty breathing, or has spells with no breathing at all (**apnea**). These are obviously serious problems that require intensive investigation in hospital. If the mother has herpes, the pediatrician needs to know in order to consider this possibility.

All of the scenarios discussed above, with the possible exception of skin sores, are nonspecific symptoms. This is the problem. So many things—some infectious, some non-infectious; some very serious, some very minor—can present themselves in exactly the same way. Herpes can cause many different things during the newborn period. Reading this section is frightening, but reading the list of symptoms from any disease can be frightening. You must realize that this problem is exceedingly unlikely to occur. It is highly preventable if you know you have herpes. Furthermore, in the unhappy event that it happens in spite of attempts at prevention, it is treatable. In fact, the problem we have with treatment is less the difficulty of finding a useful drug and *more* the delay that often occurs before the diagnosis is made. When the first sign of something serious is nonspecific, it may take days to find the correct diagnosis. Treatment is made more difficult because of the delay. If your infant becomes ill, get medical attention. You can help by making sure the physician thinks of herpes as a possibility by telling him your history. You should not use this section to make your own diagnosis. In fact, even if your baby gets all of these symptoms, herpes is unlikely. Yet it can be diagnosed only if it is specifically looked for. You can work with your physician so that the diagnosis of herpes is considered if the situation arises.

Is direct contact during delivery the only way of giving herpes to a baby?

No, but direct contact is by far the most common way of transmitting the infection. Most often, newborn herpes infection results from a lack of awareness by everyone concerned. Remember, most people (that includes pregnant women) with herpes are never aware that they have this infection. Once recurrent herpes has been diagnosed, many things can be done to prevent transmission. When it is not diagnosed, however, prevention is not possible. Take for example the case of the woman who develops primary herpes (first time ever) during the last few days or weeks of pregnancy. It is common for the primary infection to begin with nonspecific symptoms, e.g., vaginal discharge or fever or urinary discomfort. It may not show up with obvious external sores early on. The mother does not realize what is going on and therefore cannot warn the physician. Furthermore, a visual search for herpes may not be routine during labor and delivery. The exam for herpes is a visual one and includes a search for uncomfortable sores on the vaginal lips, in the perineum, around the anus, under the pubic hair, and on the cervix. The usual obstetric exam during labor, however, is a manual one—a search for the progress of labor, using the fingers, to feel the cervix. Feeling with the fingers does not detect herpes sores. The eyes detect herpes.

What can be done to prevent transmission? People in general must learn to think about herpes when vaginal discomfort or other symptoms appear during the latter part of pregnancy. Physicians who deliver babies need to make the eyes an important part of their medical tool kits during labor. In this doctor's opinion, every woman in labor, regardless of her history, should be assessed for herpes by careful examination. Some hospitals have begun to assess each woman by virus culture as well.

Another type of neonatal herpes is thought to result from infection after birth. This can come from the kiss of a parent or a nursery attendant who has either an active cold sore or a **herpetic whitlow** (herpes of the finger). Also, if another baby in the nursery has herpes, a nurse who handles the infected baby and does not wash his or her hands might pass on the virus to another infant. Infection control measures in the hospital usually prevent this.

A third type of infection mentioned previously is the one inside the womb. Happily, this occurs rarely. Probably most fetuses who get this infection early in gestation (their time inside the womb) will not survive and will be miscarried. Near term, however, it is possible (though unlikely) for little holes in the amnion (sac of waters) to open and reseal, allowing infection in. Fortunately, this is unlikely to lead to herpes infection. Herpes infection in the newborn generally occurs *during the birthing process* itself. The congenital herpes syndrome (inside the womb) does exist, however, and there is nothing that can be specifically done to prevent this type. It cannot be predicted on the basis of the type of infection or by special tests. For example, there is no greater risk for this occurring in someone with five outbreaks per month than it is for someone with one outbreak per year. In fact, why it ever happens is poorly understood.

Could I transmit herpes by kissing my baby?

The answer is yes, as described above. Remember the rules. Herpes simplex is herpes simplex. Neonatal herpes can happen with Type 1 or Type 2. Approximately one-fourth of neonatal infections are caused by Type 1. It is not actually *proven* that kissing after birth is an important source for herpes. Type 1 neonatal herpes may also result from primary Type 1 genital infection. Regardless of the mode of transmission, it is prudent to assume that kissing and other nongenital contact can cause this syndrome. We use this assumption in deciding on the safest precautions for prevention. Think of the obvious. A cold sore is herpes. A kiss from a herpes-infected mouth may be as important as a delivery through a herpes-infected vagina. This does not mean that someone with genital herpes needs to avoid kissing their newborn. You and your baby need those kisses and they are a wonderful thing. Genital herpes will not jump from your genitals to your mouth to your baby. On the other hand, if you have sores on your mouth just after the baby is born, this is a risk to be carefully dealt with during contact with the baby.

So what is done to prevent transmission after birth? First, if herpes is not active in the mother, nothing special is done. Delivery is completed normally and the baby is treated exactly like any other baby. He or she might room-in, or stay in the nursery, or both. Whatever you want to arrange with the doctor and the hospital is just fine. If herpes is *active* on the genitals when labor begins, a cesarean section is performed (more on that later). After this delivery, the baby usually should room-in with the mother or be placed in a special area of the nursery. Otherwise, things are routine. You will be advised to feed the baby in a chair and to wear a gown. The newborn baby should not be in your bed while sores are active. You need not wear a mask unless you have a sore on your mouth. You need not wear gloves unless you have a sore on your hands. You can breast-feed without problems unless you have a herpes sore on your breast. Just remember the mode of transmission. Unlike that daring young man on the flying trapeze, herpes does not fly through the air with the greatest of ease. You should not find yourself in strict isolation in the hospital because of herpes. You might find an isolation sign on your door saying "contact isolation" or "wound and skin isolation." That means your sore, if active, should be isolated while you are in hospital. Nothing else need be isolated. Most precautions in hospitals make sense. Someone should be able to explain why, or why not, you and your baby need to be isolated. Neither too little isolation nor too much isolation should occur. If your questions are not properly answered, you might ask to speak with the infection control officer (usually a nurse or physician) for an explanation.

If I get primary herpes during early pregnancy, should I have an abortion?

We have discussed the problems of primary herpes several

times in this book. If herpes were to spread into the womb, it would be more likely to occur during primary herpes, because this stage is more severe. If a fetus were to become affected early in gestation with herpes, the likelihood of miscarriage would probably be very high. A recent study by Dr. Z.A. Brown from the University of Washington described the outcome for 15 infants whose mothers had *primary* genital herpes during pregnancy. One of the five babies from mothers affected during the first trimester (12 weeks) was spontaneously miscarried and had been infected in the womb with herpes. The other four were fine. Is herpes, then, an indication for therapeutic abortion? A lot will depend on the individual's attitude toward abortion and toward the pregnancy. Even if a mother is in her eighth week and having full-bloom primary herpes, her baby's risk of getting infected in the womb is low. Exactly how low remains to be determined. The mother must decide what to do. By no stretch of the imagination is this an "accepted indication" for abortion. It is a personal decision.

In order to make the decision you must first be sure that what you had was primary and not the milder version of non-primary initial herpes, where the risk is very small. The diagnosis must be unequivocal. This means determining that the following were true:

1. it was your first ever vaginal sore like this;
2. a herpes culture test (if obtained) was positive;
3. a herpes antibody test was negative at the outset of the infection and later turned positive ("seroconversion"); and/or
4. your physician feels that your symptoms were typical for *primary* herpes (many sores involving both sides of genitals, lasting longer than 10 days and associated with fever and headache).

You should not have amniocentesis to find out anything about herpes as it can be misleading.

What, then, do I do to prevent the baby I'm carrying from contracting my herpes?

Discuss herpes with your doctor early in your pregnancy. If it is early in pregnancy, an ultrasound study might be useful later for deciding dates. In other words, when the time comes for deciding whether a cesarean section might be necessary, it is easiest if the doctor has all the available facts concerning when your baby is really due.

Learn to monitor yourself for herpes. Learn the active phases of infection. Report recurrences to your doctor.

If you have a symptomatic active recurrence during the last four to six weeks of pregnancy, see your doctor as soon as you can after the start of the recurrence. He or she should assess the sore and culture it to confirm what it is. As soon as the sore is healed, the area should be cultured again so that there is laboratory proof that the area is virus-free before electing to have a normal vaginal delivery. The new guidelines from the American College of Obstetrics and Gynecology Committee recommend that every woman with a history of genital herpes have at least one negative culture before labor (with no subsequent new symptoms of active herpes) before deciding on the normal route of delivery. Yet doing weekly cultures near term without symptoms seemed to be a poor method for prevention of infection in one study from California. These investigators also found that neonatal herpes is extremely unlikely to occur, even if the mother with recurrent herpes is culture-positive during labor! The best way to prevent prenatal herpes, therefore, is an area of academic controversy. I recommend that your doctor carefully examine with a strong light source the external genitals (those parts shown in Figure 8B on page 43) as a part of your last two or three prenatal visits and once again during labor. A virus culture, using one moistened swab of all of the external genital areas, should be taken on at least one of the prenatal visits and repeated during labor. This will let your doctor know what your normal genital skin looks like so that he or she will be fairly confident that the appearance is normal during labor before electing to assist with a normal vaginal delivery. If a sore or symptoms of a sore are present at labor, a **cesarean section** is indicated. If all looks well, and the last virus culture is negative, a cesarean is not required.

Unless a very important reason exists for needing one, a fetal scalp monitor should probably be *avoided* if you have a history of herpes.

Obtain a cesarean section, if and only if you have *active* herpes or if you have just had active herpes that your doctor thinks might not be healed when you go into labor. A decision about healing can be a tough one. Essentially we are considering the active phases (Chapter 3) as active and the inactive as inactive. Because of the high stakes involved in pregnancy, something a bit more than usual is tacked on at the end of an outbreak as an extra measure of safety. A culture is especially useful in keeping the time to a minimum. If the episode near the end of term is a *primary* herpes, it would be wise to extend the safety period even further. *Primary* herpes in late pregnancy should be managed by a physician. Careful monitoring and/or antiviral treatment may be indicated.

Once membranes rupture, if herpes is active, an urgent cesarean section is indicated. This operation can be more leisurely arranged during labor if membranes are intact. If the herpes is not active, a cesarean is not necessary because of herpes.

Does a cesarean delivery always prevent transmission?

Because herpes is generally transmitted by direct contact, when a physical barrier remains between a herpes sore and a baby's skin (the barrier is the sac of waters), the risk of neonatal infection is extremely small. Thus, bypassing an active sore by delivering the baby through the abdomen (cesarean section) will not allow the direct spread of the infection. This is an extremely effective method of prevention. Whether you will need a cesarean section or not will depend upon whether you happen to be in the midst of a herpes recurrence (active phase of infection) when labor begins. The statistical likelihood of needing a cesarean section will depend upon how often you get recurrences. As far as we know, your recurrence frequency rate will not affect the risk to your baby. It will only affect your chances of needing a cesarean section.

Once the sac of waters barrier is broken, the possibility of direct transmission to the baby becomes more likely. If this occurs without your knowing it (there may be small holes that heal up without symptoms), then a cesarean section might not prevent infection. The practical risk of this causing problems in your baby is very small indeed.

Confusion might arise when the bag of waters breaks (leaky fluid is usually obvious, but sudden clear fluid discharges in late pregnancy need checking out at a hospital). Once the membranes rupture—and this may be the first symptom of labor—it is only a matter of time until an active herpes on the outside gets to the inside. This is because the barrier is broken and a **wet path** has developed. In other words, there is a fluid connection from outside to inside held nicely at body temperature, allowing the virus to find its way inside. If herpes is active on the skin when the membranes rupture, it is only a matter of time before the virus gets to the baby. Therefore, cesarean section has to be done immediately. Some confusion has arisen recently, suggesting that it is all right to wait four hours from the time membranes rupture until the cesarean section is performed. This is not true. A cesarean section should be performed the minute that preparations can be made if herpes is considered to be active at the time the membranes rupture.

In summary, cesarean section does prevent herpes transmission to the newborn when *recurrent* herpes is active and membranes have not been ruptured for a prolonged period of time. This holds for almost all situations that might arise if everyone involved, from mother to physician, is thinking of herpes and ready to handle each situation thoughtfully.

Why don't all pregnant women with genital herpes have a cesarean section?

There is often a feeling among some mothers with herpes that cesarean is the way to go regardless of the situation. Often this stems from the burden of potential guilt that the mother feels would arise from an infection in the baby. This is a very noble thought indeed. Unfortunately it is often based upon a lack of understanding of the facts. Here are the facts:

1. Genital herpes is a common problem, while neonatal herpes is an uncommon problem.
2. When necessary, a cesarean section may need to be performed for active herpes during labor. When herpes is inactive, however, cesarean section offers no advantages over normal vaginal delivery.
3. Despite its overall good safety record, the risk of cesarean section to the mother is actually much higher than that of vaginal delivery. After all, cesarean birth is a form of surgery. It means a longer hospital stay and a higher risk of postpartum (after birth) complications such as fever and infection. The risk of cesarean section is low, yet the risks of surgery clearly outweigh any potential benefits when herpes is not active at the time of labor.
4. Even cesarean section won't necessarily prevent neonatal herpes, which may come from other sources than the mother's genital herpes—for example, transmission of herpes from Aunt Sadie's fever blister. It is much better to think out the problem and use care in avoiding transmission. A panacea prevention may just confuse the issues.

Is there treatment for an affected baby?

Yes. Antiviral treatment in general will be discussed in Chapter 11. You may find more specific information there. Newer antiviral chemicals have made drug treatment for active herpes a reality. We now have very effective means of killing the virus while it is active. Our problems, in general, in devising new ways to kill herpes are twofold. First, therapy cannot undo damage already done to vital structures, although it can probably stop progression of damage from the infection. Second, it does not alter latent infection (see Chapter 1), and therefore virus infection may recur. Suspected neonatal herpes should be quickly and aggressively diagnosed. If a newborn baby becomes ill and the mother has a history of herpes, she should make sure that the pediatrician knows of her history. If the father or any other sexual partner has herpes, that also may be important since the mother could then have herpes without knowing it. Remember, too, that herpes can occur even where both parents deny any history of ever having had a herpes sore. Make sure someone explains to you how the possibilities of herpes (and other problems) are being investigated. If herpes is not a consideration to the physician, is that because there is a good reason not to consider it? It is certainly possible to have good medical reasons not to consider the diagnosis of herpes in a newborn, but you should suggest looking for herpes just to make sure that your doctor has thought of the possibility. If herpes is not a possibility, your physician will explain why it is not.

Adenine arabinoside (ara-A, Vira-A®) and acyclovir (Zovirax®) are both very useful agents for treating neonatal herpes. Neither agent can reverse damage already done, however. Happily, physicians are diagnosing neonatal herpes more quickly. Still, the diagnosis is often made after damage is done. We need to focus on prevention—but prevention is needed most where it is applied the least, i.e., where the mother does *not* think she has genital herpes.

Occasionally a baby will be treated with acyclovir when there is no illness whatsoever. The theoretical situation would be after a normal vaginal delivery or prolonged membrane rupture when, at that point, it is discovered the baby was already exposed. This could happen when the sore is noticed after delivery or in the unlikely event of asymptomatic virus shedding. After telling you that no scientific studies have been performed to support the use of acyclovir in this setting, and after adding that many experts in this field prefer *not* to use the drug in this setting, I will state that I tend to prescribe acyclovir in this situation. It is my prejudice that preventing herpes from starting (if that is possible with a drug) is far superior to treating it once it is there. Furthermore, when you analyze all the data, this agent seems to be pretty safe.

If I have active herpes during labor, may I still have epidural anesthesia?

Yes, unless your herpes is a true primary. In that situation, there is a slight risk of herpes meningitis (see Chapter 3), which *might* cause complications from the epidural. In that very unusual setting, the anesthetist may wish to opt for a general anesthetic during the cesarean section. Because of this *theoretical risk,* some anesthetists have opted for general anesthetic even during recurrent episodes of genital herpes. Recurrent herpes has never been associated in any way with any proven risk increase after epidural anesthesia. In fact, Drs. Sheth, Ramanathan, Durtzman, and Turndorf reported their results from the New York University Medical Center at the International Anesthesia Research Society Meetings in March of 1985. They studied 56 patients in labor with genital herpes infection. Despite the fact that 33 of these women had epidural anesthesia, no complications related to the anesthetic developed in either group.

Active recurrent or inactive recurrent genital herpes is not a contraindication to epidural anesthesia.

What are my baby's chances of getting herpes?

Neonatal herpes is very unlikely to occur in an infant born to a mother who has genital herpes and knows that she has it. By contrast, when the mother does not know she has genital herpes, and especially when the infection is occurring for the first time during labor, her baby is at much greater risk. A mother with *recurrent* infection is unlikely to transmit infection for the following reasons:

- She has a greater than 99 percent chance of knowing on the basis of her symptoms whether she is going to be culture-positive and potentially exposing the baby. If symptoms of an active phase of infection are present, she will be able to obtain a cesarean section.
- If she is shedding virus without symptoms, the chances are that this virus will be coming from an external area and only contact the baby for a short time, if at all.

- Because she has recurrent infection, she is likely to have high levels of anti-herpes antibody that will be passed on to the baby and the amniotic fluid surrounding the baby, thereby neutralizing the virus in most cases before it has a chance to get into the epithelial cells of the newborn infant.
- Most infants who are exposed to the virus will never actually acquire infection, for the reasons listed above. Of those who do, the vast majority will never develop disease as a result.
- If exposure to virus has occurred, the physician has the choice of treating the infant with a very effective antiviral agent, acyclovir (oral or intravenous). Because the chances of the baby getting sick are so low, even after a positive exposure, many physicians will elect not to treat the baby. This is an area of academic controversy. I favor treatment before disease develops, in an attempt to prevent this from happening, although I recognize that no clinical trials have been performed to examine this question from a scientific point of view.

Physicians must make an educated guess about the actual risk of any mother with recurrent genital herpes giving birth to a baby with a herpes infection since no accurate statistics exist. In my opinion, the risk is less than 1 chance in 5,000 that this will happen to any individual with recurrent genital herpes so long as the usual guidelines are followed. This makes the risk of herpes no greater than the risk for a variety of other congenital diseases, and herpes should not prevent you from having children should you elect to do so.

By contrast, where an infant is born to a mother having a primary genital herpes infection during labor, vaginal delivery may be associated with as much as a 50 percent risk of infection in the infant. *Primary* herpes occuring any time in the third trimester of pregnancy is associated with significant risk to the baby. Recognizing that no trials have tested the question, in *primary* genital herpes of the third trimester, I would treat the mother with intravenous and/or oral acyclovir for 10 days and then deliver the baby by cesarean section at full term (nine months).

7

HERPES AND CANCER

Who cares about your questions, you still won't be going back home. You may as well give back your glasses. And your pajamas.
ALEKSANDR SOLZHENITSYN,
Cancer Ward

What evidence seems to show that herpes causes cancer?

Because there is no proof that herpes simplex is a cause of cancer, one must examine the circumstantial evidence that suggests that cancer and herpes might be related. After all the evidence is in, you will find that a scientific argument about the causes of cervical cancer still exists. The association between herpes and cancer is not nearly as certain, for example, as the relationship between smoking and cancer.

The first piece of evidence is that sex causes **cervical cancer.** Cancer of the cervix is a common tumor in prostitutes, rare in Catholic nuns. It occurs more often in women who experience their first sexual contact early and who have more sexual partners in their lifetime. It should not be surprising, then, to find that one sexually transmitted agent, namely herpes simplex, is more common in women with cervical cancer than in those without. About 15 years ago studies began to show, over and over again, a **seroepidemiologic** association between the two diseases. In other words, a blood, or serum ("sero-"), test for herpes antibodies, (specifically antibodies to herpes simplex Type 2), would show up more often in groups of women ("-epidemiologic") *with* cancer than in groups without. By themselves, however, these studies tell us little. We already know that sex is associated with cervical cancer. We are also virtually certain that sex predisposes an individual to getting genital herpes. So why the surprise when both herpes and cancer of the cervix were found to be more common in women who have more sex-related risk factors? It would have been more surprising *not* to find this. We *still don't know* if the real cause of cervical cancer is herpes or some other "male factor." Among the other suspect causes being actively investigated:

1. **Chlamydia trachomatis.** In men this may cause **urethritis** (NGU or NSU) and in women **pelvic inflammatory disease** (PID). It may also cause **cervicitis** (inflammation of the cervix) and abdominal discomfort in women. It has also been linked to one cause of urinary discomfort called the **acute urethral syndrome.**

2. **Sperm.** If a male factor is important in causing cervical cancer, why not one that is nearly universal? It has been suggested that the DNA (hereditary material) in sperm may somehow associate itself with cells from the cervix, causing a change to a common cell. Another conjecture is that proteins on the surface of a sperm head may lead to cancerous mutations.

3. **Wart virus.** The **human papillomavirus** (HPV), known to cause venereal warts, has also been called an **oncogenic** (cancer-causing) virus. This virus is almost certainly the true cervical cancer virus. Certain subtypes are very closely related to cancer development. This is a very exciting area of research now, which is likely to yield many specific answers in the near future.

4. **Smegma.** This is the name for the slightly sticky collection of secretion fluids and sloughed skin cells, sometimes with a characteristic odor, which may be found under the foreskin of the penis. The association of smegma with cancer stems almost entirely from the low statistical evidence of cervical

cancer in women of the traditional Jewish faith, whose partners are likely to have been circumcized.

A host of other agents including **Trichomonas vaginalis** and **cytomegalovirus**, have been suggested as possible causes for cervical cancer. Continued research may provide some answers.

Aside from the seroepidemiologic association, some other evidence suggests that herpes might be a possible cause of cancer. Herpes simplex virus can, under special laboratory conditions, cause a cell to change character. That is, a normal cell taken from a hamster and treated with herpes in a special way has been known to form a cancerous tumor when reintroduced into the hamster's body. Certain parts of herpes viruses can be detected in some human cervical tumors using special tests called **nucleic acid probes.** Some investigators claim that herpes antibodies can actually be used in certain circumstances to determine how well a cervical cancer is responding to treatment. Furthermore, herpes can be made to cause cancer in laboratory animals under the correct conditions.

Meanwhile, as we get better and better at detecting and probing for causes, it is clear that invasive cancer of the cervix is becoming less and less common. Early Pap smear changes are often treated so quickly that cancer is never allowed to develop. In fact, some would say we treat Pap smear abnormalities too quickly, since often they get better by themselves.

While human papillomavirus is quickly replacing herpes simplex as the most likely cause of cervical cancer, the Pap smear is still an important health tool for any sexually active woman. Cervical cancer is unlikely to develop, and an abnormality is very easy to detect before it becomes cancerous. If cancer does develop, it starts out very slowly, allowing lots of time to take successful curative action during the early stages. The Pap smear is used for detection—use it regularly.

One other cancer is associated with herpes: cancer of the **vulva,** the woman's external genitals. This is also a slow-growing cancer, which is much less common than cancer of the cervix. Its association with herpes is also confusing. The symptoms are commonly external itching or pain, or the observance of a growth. Its most common locations—on the external genitals—parallel those of genital herpes. Although itching of the vaginal area is seldom related to cancer, persistent vaginal itching should be explored for possible causes. See your physician if you are concerned.

If I have herpes, is it on the cervix? Inside the vagina?

During primary genital herpes, 9 out of 10 women with herpes on the labia also have herpes on the cervix. Sometimes this may cause **cervicitis,** or inflammation of the cervix with an associated vaginal discharge. Sores can develop on the cervix as well. Herpes is probably a cause of nonspecific cervicitis more often than is realized. Cervicitis and discharge are common during primary herpes, even in the absence of external sores—sometimes because external sores develop a bit later in the course of infection and sometimes because external sores never develop during primary herpes.

Involvement of the internal genitals (cervix) in recurrent herpes is quite another matter. A carefully performed study has shown that herpes might be recovered from the cervix in only four percent of recurrent cases. In fact, it may be that many of these were not really on the cervix, but may have appeared to be there because of an artifact in the test, caused by the "wet path" that exists between cervix and sore. If a sore is just near to the entrance to the vagina, then one must come so close to it on the way in to examine the cervix that a positive culture may result from virus innocently passing by. Internal infection with herpes is by no means the rule—genital herpes is an external infection for the most part. It occurs mainly on the vaginal lips, the perianal area, the perineum (between anus and vagina) and the pubic region in women. The cervix is an uncommon site of infection during recurrences.

What are my chances, then, of getting cervical cancer?

There are different types of cervical cancer according to both epidemiologists who look at the problem and to the women affected by this disease. Cancer detected on a Pap smear before any damage whatsoever is done to the person occurs in about 1 in 1,000 women over the age of 20. Depending upon the study you believe, the risk increases to 2 to 8 per 1,000 women with genital herpes. Clinically significant cervical cancer (one that has gone far enough that it might do harm to the person if not dealt with immediately) occurs with much less frequency (closer to 7 or 8 of 100,000 women over the age of 20). The risk of this type of cancer occurring after genital herpes is diagnosed is increased to approximately 15 to 100 cases per 100,000 women over the age of 20. The average age of occurrence is in a woman's late forties, although cervical cancer can be seen as early as the teens or as late as the eighties.

What should I do to prevent cervical cancer from becoming a problem?

A **Pap smear** is a simple procedure and can become a part of your annual gynecological examination. It is quick and simple to do correctly. The best time to have it done (or to do it yourself if you've learned how) is just before or at ovulation, when estrogen hormone levels are high. This means the cells are flatter and easier to interpret under the microscope. The test can also be done at any other time if ovulation is an inconvenient time to make the visit to the physician. First, a plastic or metal speculum is inserted into the vagina, as pictured in Figure 17. This allows the examiner to see the cervix by gently pushing the walls of the vagina aside. Any vaginal discharge and cervical mucus coating the cervix are then swabbed away using a cotton swab. A wooden scraper, shaped like a stretched popsicle stick and made for this purpose, is used to painlessly scrape the cells from the surface of the cervix onto a slide, which is then sent to the laboratory.

The Pap smear will detect any unusual cells from the cervix. If cells are cancerous, it will detect them. If cells are just upset from infection, it will detect them also. All of these cells will be called **abnormal.** Since cancer of the cervix is very slow to grow, a regular (yearly) Pap smear will be an adequate test. Some physicians feel that even fewer Pap smears are needed. As long as they stay normal—Class 1—one per year is plenty. If your Pap smear is abnormal in any way, more frequent smears may be appropriate. Discuss this with your physician.

Whether you have herpes or not, the yearly Pap smear is a good idea. Rest assured that if you follow this regimen, you will detect any cancer of the cervix while it is 100 percent curable. I recommend putting this cancer out of your mind except for one big red mark on each new calendar—the day for your yearly Pap test.

My Pap smear is abnormal. What does that mean?

The Pap smear is a method of examining the cells that line your

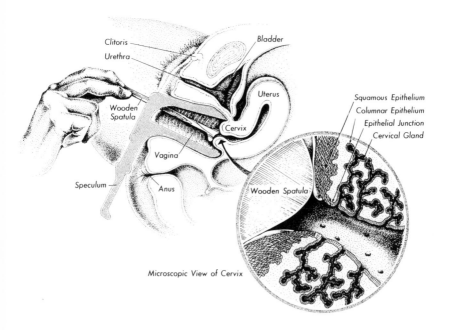

17. *The Pap smear being taken by the health practitioner. The wooden stick samples the cells of the cervix (insert), which are then placed onto a glass microscope slide. A person called a cytologist examines the cells under the microscope to see if they look the way they are supposed to look.*

cervix. Anything that changes those cells will change your Pap smear. During primary herpes, a Pap smear will be abnormal from infection but will change back to normal after the primary episode has cleared; this abnormal smear is of no concern. Other infections may also change the Pap smear, such as **trichomoniasis, Gardnerella vaginitis,** and **gonorrhea.** In each case, if the Pap has become abnormal as a symptom of infection, treatment of the infection will cause the Pap to revert to normal eventually. A Pap will also be abnormal if cancer of the cervix has developed. It is obviously quite important to find out if your abnormal Pap is from infection or cancer. How is this done?

Pap abnormalities are classified. The classifications will vary from city to city, state to state, province to province, and country to country. There are "scores" ranging from normal to obvious invasive cancer, with many gray areas in between. When your score is normal, regardless of where you live, a little celebration is in order, along with a mental note to repeat the process in a year. When the score is abnormal, there are several things to do. If the most severely abnormal condition is detected, indicating invasive cancer, a **colposcopy** is generally performed (see next page). If less severely abnormal scores are discovered, your best bet is first to make sure that all possible infections have been ruled out. Your doctor will do (or may already have done) a culture test for **Chlamydia,** gonorrhea, **Candida,** and Gardnerella. An examination for **Trichomonas vaginalis** is also performed. If your abnormal Pap was taken during or shortly after your primary herpes, you may also want to repeat the test to see if the situation has improved on its own. If another infection is present, get your Pap repeated two or three months later to see if it has returned to normal. Your doctor will help you sort that out.

Now, let's say that you still have an abnormal test. You've had your infection treated, if one was present. You've waited several months. If the score shows only a mild abnormality, you will likely be advised to wait and see and to have another test in a few months. Probably this abnormal score will eventually vanish. If your score shows consistently abnormal cells, you may be sent for a **colposcopy test.** This is an examination of the cervix much like the Pap smear. The speculum exam is repeated, as for the Pap smear. Then, a microscope-like instrument is inserted through the speculum, giving the physician a very close look at the surface of the cervix. Biopsies are taken for further laboratory examination. A cervix biopsy may feel like a pinch or may feel like nothing at all. The procedure is very, very safe and a small amount of bleeding is to be expected. The laboratory will examine these biopsies and offer an opinion. If invasive or microinvasive cancer is present on the biopsy, the therapy is removal of the cancer. This may require surgery, but not always. The most common surgical course taken is called a **cone biopsy,** in which only the inner core of the cervix is removed through the vagina. Generally, a cone biopsy does not prevent you from experiencing a normal pregnancy.

The different possible therapies to be chosen at this point are beyond the scope of this book. If your biopsy fits a less severe category, you enter a gray zone where arguments exist about what therapy you should have. You might be advised in one center to have a cone biopsy for severe dysplasia and in another center to wait, see, and repeat for *carcinoma in situ.* Why all the confusion? Most women in this gray area actually will not progress to invasive cancer, if left alone. Many patients will revert to a normal condition with no intervention —however, many physicians will argue that most is not good enough.

The safest (and most serious) thing to do with cervical tissue diagnosed as being in a gray area is to remove it from the cervix. Have you ever been asked if you see the proverbial glass of water as "half full or half empty"? The right course of action is not cast in stone—everyone is looking for answers, and if the situation should arise for you, discuss it at length with your doctor and read a lot more on the topic. Remember this, however: if you have been told that you have an abnormal result from a routine Pap smear, you have found the problem early and can get treatment that is 100 percent effective and safe!

8

THE PSYCHOLOGY
OF HERPES

*Yet it is hardly possible to take up one's residence in the kingdom of
the ill unprejudiced by the lurid metaphors with which it has been
landscaped.*
SUSAN SONTAG,
Illness as Metaphor

What emotional impact does herpes have on people?

Remember that a herpes infection may cause a spectrum of
physical distress ranging from asymptomatic (no symptoms) to
very severe. Just as the physical symptoms of herpes are not
the same for everyone, so the emotional impact of herpes is
also variable. It cannot be typified, categorized, or com-
partmentalized. If you have herpes, the emotional effect on you
will obviously depend to some extent on how severely it affects
you physically. A painful and prolonged primary infection might
certainly result in a severe reaction of shock and anger. Any
emotional reaction will also depend upon how you were informed of the diagnosis. Was the person knowledgeable?
Judgmental? Informative? What were your preconceived no-
tions? Had you learned about herpes before it happened and
prepared yourself for the possibility, or had you thought, "It
could never happen to me!"? Is your background a religious
one? Had you believed that herpes was a punishment visited on
those who have it? Have you known others with herpes? What

were their reactions to herpes, emotional and physical? What have been their experiences with this infection? Can you accept the inevitable generally, or more specifically about herpes? Do you feel guilt or shame about the circumstances under which you received the infection? Do you feel hurt by the person who transmitted herpes to you? Do you know how you got it? Has herpes interrupted your lifestyle? By how much? Are you afraid of getting involved because you will have to tell your partner?

All the possible scenarios of reactions would more than fill this chapter. Some of the more common reactions to herpes are listed below. Some may be only temporary, while others may have lasting impact for the individual. You should not necessarily expect to feel *any* of these things. Rather, you *should* realize that you are not alone with your feelings, whatever they may be.

On first learning about herpes, you may have a feeling of **shock.** There might be a sudden change in the image you have of your own body, or a sense of loss. Some people react with panic upon hearing the word "herpes," which they associate with other words such as "contagious" and "incurable." You might feel this, for example, during a severe primary infection, when you are ill and terribly uncomfortable. You might have been told you have herpes, but informed of little else. You might have heard that herpes is painful or incurable, and might imagine (incorrectly) either that this primary herpes will recur with the same intensity or that it will go on forever.

Shock may also be your response if the diagnosis has been unexpected. You may have gone to the doctor because of something like a recurring yeast infection, hemorrhoids, or a spider bite, only to be told you have genital herpes. You may feel trapped inside a defective body over which you feel you have lost control. Regaining emotional and physical control requires regrouping your thoughts. Adjusting to having herpes cannot be instantaneous. It comes through experience, study, and observation. After all, any major change in life requires a period of adjustment. I would stress the term "normalization." People with herpes should be striving toward that goal. The normalization process requires the passage of time—time to gain perspective. Normalization comes through an active process of learning the facts about herpes and, just as importantly, passing *through* the stage of self-pity toward an ability to work with those facts.

At first the diagnosis of herpes may be **frightening,** because of the possibilities of cancer or problems with future pregnancies or future romances. Think back: we were the vaccinated generation, the children of the penicillin era. Marcus Welby, M.D., never failed to cure our diseases, no matter how serious. Everyone knows that "you could be hit by a bus while crossing the street," but nobody thinks it will happen, not really. Everyone knows that herpes is the "disease of the 80s," but nobody expects to get it—much in the way that VD has been something that *other* people get. You may have feared getting herpes and now you may fear having it. Yet upon having it and understanding it, one can see that the physical symptoms do not threaten your life or sanity. Nor does the physical distress of herpes have to threaten your health. You can certainly be sexually healthy, physically healthy, mentally healthy, and spiritually healthy *while you have herpes*.

Until the facts are clear, your own **fear** may well be the dominant emotional reaction to your herpes. It may be difficult to relate to others while you are afraid. There may be a desire to seek out unrealistic cures rather than to face the issues directly. This may arise in part from the difficulty of finding material to read that does not scare you even more. Alternatively, you may have come across literature that reassures you beyond believability. You may not have yet located a health practitioner who has explained the details of herpes to you. Herpes is a well-characterized, recurrent viral infection, which you can fully understand. Being in possession of all the facts will help put things into perspective.

You may feel **shame** about having a "social disease." This may be amplified by the jokes of your friends or by the expressions of their own fears. A feeling may predominate that there is something shameful to hide. In fact, you may not wish to discuss herpes with some people. Herpes is like any other secret. Because its origin and domain is in the sexual act, you may feel strongly about keeping herpes a secret—private, discreet. This might reflect how you feel about the sexual encounter that you feel resulted in herpes. However, anxieties which may arise because you are keeping the secret should be distinguished in your mind from any feeling of shame *for having acquired herpes*. Whom you tell is up to you. Some people feel the need to talk about herpes to casual friends. This may make things feel more acceptable to you or it might give you an ally to condone the situation. But do not rely on other people to give you your peace of mind. Confession does not solve the problem. Occasionally, if circumstances dictate, confession of some kind may be appropriate, even necessary. For instance, you may need to clear the air and discuss the details of a love affair because having herpes has made it difficult *not* to discuss those. A religious person may feel the need for absolution. Any confession will be based on individual needs and individual circumstances. One confesses the deed, however, not the virus.

It is critical that we separate the deed from the virus. Good deeds or bad, right deeds or wrong, happy deeds or sad, these definitions are left to the philosopher and the theologian.[1] The moral choices are left to the individual. Viruses are another matter. Viruses are in the realm of the virologist, the physician, and the epidemiologist. Viruses do not make moral choices. We accept them as "bad" because they cause sores and are parasitic. However, viruses do not choose on whom they land on the basis of moral principles. For instance, a virus called polio can paralyze children. Before the advent of polio vaccine 25 years ago, countless thousands of children were paralyzed each year. There was nothing moral or immoral about this phenomenon, however; it was simply the result of the nature of the virus combined with the susceptibility of children. In that vein, herpes may be passed by contact from the mouth of a mother to the eye of her child because of the most innocent and morally correct act that the mind could imagine— a loving kiss. Herpes sores on the genitals of an adult, then,

[1]Inspired by parallels drawn by Thomas Szasz in his book *Sex by Prescription* (New York: Penguin Books, 1980).

should not be seen as an issue of morality. Shame may be appropriate in one circumstance and inappropriate in another. Yet it has nothing to do with the biological facts related to this virus.

Alternatively, a feeling of **guilt** may result from the nature of the sexual involvement. You may also feel guilty because of your potential to transmit herpes—a problem minimized by education and awareness, and by open and frank discussions with sexual partners. Ironically, people with herpes occasionally find themselves in the position of soothing the guilt of the partner who transmitted the infection.

Anger is a common reaction to herpes. Initial feelings of shock or the subsequent feelings of guilt may give way to anger. Anger is a normal response to a loss. Herpes has invaded your domain. Even though you know that active phases follow a cycle, you are faced with accepting the fact that the virus itself is not possible to eradicate—a feeling that can turn to frustration.

Anger may also be directed at the person who transmitted the infection to you; you may feel tainted or betrayed or compromised; perhaps you even feel abandoned. The fact is that while the rare person with serious underlying emotional disturbances might purposefully transmit herpes to others, the overwhelming majority of people who transmit herpes will fall into one of these categories:

- They did not know what the sores (or cuts, or slits, or pimples, or whatever) were.
- They never had any symptoms suggestive of herpes.
- They knew about the presence of herpes but were mistaken about the active phases of infection.
- They showed the sores to a health practitioner and were told they were nothing to worry about.
- They were tested for herpes and the virus culture was negative, and they did not understand what this meant.
- They understood the active phases of infection, were careful, and still transmitted the infection.

Most situations are like one of the first five, and none of the six categories describe evil people, with "malice afore-thought." Though conscientious, a careful person with herpes may have been told that herpes was "just a virus infection" or "just a cold sore of the genitals." They may not have realized the need to avoid transmission. In fact, most partners of persons who have just contracted primary genital herpes deny any history of herpes. This is not because the partners are liars. Symptoms may never have suggested to the individual that herpes may be present. Furthermore, many people are misinformed. Even the person who knew about his or her herpes infection, but failed to tell, may not have had the courage or known enough medical information to properly explain the problem. Perhaps he or she felt inarticulate or shy, or was afraid to tamper with the relationship. Possibly the first time they told a partner, it resulted in a traumatic breakup. He or she is in a confusing position, with a tough responsibility. If you find yourself temporarily despising the person who gave you the herpes, vent your anger in other ways. If you are sure who gave you herpes, inform, but try not to hurt, this person, since this would be useless. It could also be later regretted. It may be a difficult time for your partner also. Often anger directed at the person who you think gave you herpes may result from misunderstanding about how transmission might occur. Later you might find yourself turning your anger inward for being "foolish" enough to catch herpes. This is a more destructive form of anger. If you are angry at a friend, the friend can walk away, but it is more difficult to walk away from yourself. Try to place your anger correctly in the lap of the *virus*. In other words, remember that distinction between *virus* and *deed*. Be aware that herpes is a reality among people in the 1980s who make love, a reality that encompasses those who are rich or poor, clean or unkempt, "cool" or not.

Your anger might also be directed at the person who informs you of the diagnosis—the health professional. He or she is also the one who fails to offer you a cure, and this may be seen as the worst "sin" of all. Every physician or health care professional must be prepared for this. If the physician's answers to patients' questions are thoughtful and informed, much anger and frustration will be minimized. When the physician makes the mistake of sitting in judgment or of offering inadequate information, anger directed against the physician can be expected.

Depression is a common emotional reaction to herpes. Many people are understandably depressed by having the infection. Anyone would rather not have herpes if that were possible. Depression may result from the frustration of having an "incurable" disease. A sense of hopelessness will arise in some people with each active recurrence. Very frequent recurrences may have someone who is angry or depressed cycling in and out of these emotions while trying to cope with the actual physical distress of the recurrences. It is normal to feel depressed over having herpes. It would be a sign of not caring for yourself and others, or just plain stupidity, not to feel sad over the change of life that herpes may impose on you. You now have an obligation to discuss herpes with sexual partners, to become aware of your recurrence patterns and avoid sore contact during active phases, and to monitor childbirth. This means some loss of spontaneity and freedom. Depression may also result from a loss of self-esteem—a feeling that you will never be perfect or that you have not lived up to your expectations. And whether it is fear of transmission or concern over the temporary discoloration of skin, the self-esteem we have tied up in our sexuality is very real. Sexual acts leave the participants vulnerable. When herpes complicates this vulnerability, there may be a tendency to feel wronged. A feeling of isolation may follow. Isolation, after all, can protect from further losses. Isolation carried to its extreme, however, can result in a self-imposed "sexual leper" effect: in other words, the feeling that one is alone and *should* be alone, for protection as well as for self-punishment.

There is a point, for some people, when depression becomes overwhelming, when a healthy degree of sadness changes to an overbearing feeling of hopelessness. At this point, depression becomes a problem of its own quite separate from herpes. It may be difficult to tell where the predictable feelings about an upsetting thing like herpes end and where **clinical depression** begins. This is an unusual reaction to herpes, however. If it does occur, clinical depression may make you feel as if life's efforts are futile. Most (but not all) people who are clinically depressed will feel "blue" or low, so low that it becomes increasingly difficult to enjoy life, to have good times. The appetite may decrease (or occasionally increase) with weight loss (or weight gain). Commonly, people who are depressed will feel a loss of their normal body energy and vitality. Sleep patterns may be interrupted by difficulty falling asleep (tossing and turning) or by awakening in the middle of the night and not being able to get back to sleep. Depression may also lead to loss of the usual "drive" at work. Sexual desire may disappear. It may become difficult to concentrate. There may be thoughts of suicide—there may even be a plan for how to commit suicide. Other manifestations of clinical depression might be aches and pains that turn out to have no physical cause or phobias—fear of heights or fear of closed spaces, for example. If symptoms of depression take on importance of their own in your life, apart from herpes—especially if several of these symptoms occur together—then you owe it to yourself to treat the depression seriously. Clinical depression can happen to anyone, with herpes or not, and should not go unchecked. If you think you might be clinically depressed, it is treatable— seek help.

Can my emotions trigger a recurrence?

Triggers for herpes are discussed in Chapter 3. The acknowledged triggers are all different types of stressors (anything that causes stress, whether good or bad). Those stressors can include such things as menstrual periods or surgery or excessive sunlight. Most people feel that one stressor or another is responsible for triggering *some* recurrences. However, the overwhelming majority of herpes recurrences in any one individual happen for no apparent reason. They occur without relation to stressors and without changes in immunity. Recurrences just *happen*. Under careful analysis, there is a suggestion that people who are undergoing a high degree of emotional stress *may* have more recurrences than those who are not. However, there are numerous factors that may interact at any moment to trigger a recurrence, and they are difficult to categorize or control.

There has never been any scientific evidence to suggest that learning to diminish emotional stressors will diminish herpes recurrences—or for that matter alter your chances of having a heart attack or of getting an ulcer. Every effort should be made, however, to take control of the stressors in your changing life, not because you can count on a reduction in herpes recurrences, but because life is, by its nature, a series of stressful events of which herpes infection is one. There is a great tendency in newspapers and magazines to make stress control and coping with herpes seem synonymous. This is not based in fact but rather in the *hope* that new stress control methods may help to diminish recurrences of herpes. Unfortunately this may have a boomerang effect whereby guilt develops when herpes recurs. A feeling of recurring failure can develop: "Why couldn't I prevent this one? What have I done wrong?" A straight cause-and-effect relation between emotional stress and herpes is not realistic. Furthermore, herpes is a very strong stressor in its own right. Stress control and coping methods are useful means of living with herpes. If you find that certain types of stress controls also become useful for you in keeping your recurrence rate low, then you are among the lucky.

What can I do to cope?

Follow these rules or replace them with reasonable alternatives of your own:

1. Go to a clinic or your own doctor for diagnosis (see Chapter 4). Believe it or not, you will have your distress partially relieved by *knowing*. If you know for sure that you have herpes, you can deal with it in a logical and straightforward fashion.

2. You are not alone with your herpes, and you are not alone with your feelings. Realize that your emotional response, whether it be shock or anger, is something others have also experienced.
3. Face your fears directly. Expect certain aspects of herpes to bother you more than others and learn more about those aspects.
4. Be realistic. Researching herpes for the sake of knowledge and in order for you to regain control over your own life is a goal to be applauded. You will *not,* however, find a cure by frantically reading all the latest literature. Hoping for a cure is fine. It is critical that a cure be sought, that an effective method for prevention be sought, and that improved treatment be found. These will not come, however, from panic or fear. A cure for herpes may become a reality, eventually. For now, establish an easy method for keeping up with the latest in herpes research so that good treatments come to your attention.
5. Avoid discussions about your herpes with casual friends and acquaintances. The facts about your herpes need to be shared with someone else if the following are true:
   • If sharing the information will help you in some important way. For example, tell your doctor so that he or she can make sure you have herpes or tell members of a self-help group with whom you might share similar personal experiences. You may also choose to share the information with a close friend. This is a personal decision. Some people choose never to tell friends. They lose in some ways, but they diminish the risks inherent in "going public."
   • If sharing the information will help someone else in some important way. For example, tell your present and future sexual partners, a friend who has herpes, etc.
   • If you choose to tell a friend with whom you have no sexual intimacy or plans for sexual intimacy, think about who might be the right person in advance. Avoid telling casual acquaintances. Ask for confidentiality; you should

feel confident that this person will respect your wishes. Explain to this friend that you want to avoid pity. The last thing you need is someone to feel sorry for you. If you feel that you would benefit from having someone close to talk to about herpes, search out an equal who will not use the information for a "superiority trip," but who will be able to offer personal advice and criticism. The right friend will not pity you, but rather will help you to avoid self-pity.

6. Try to avoid making your herpes the subject of others' gossip. Gossip is painful and useless, but it is a social fact. It stems from ignorance. Herpes is a "juicy story," and you are best off not becoming the subject. You may not wish to mention your herpes casually or socially. It is simply not anyone else's business, unless you plan to have sexual contact with that person.

7. Sort out your thoughts concerning the telling of sexual partners. (More of this a little later.)

8. If your anger is a problem for you, make sure that you seek and find logical and acceptable answers to your questions. Participate actively in finding those answers, and get herpes into perspective. *Herpes is not you.* It is, however, a reality in your life. In other words, if you are pregnant, make sure that the person scheduled to follow your pregnancy and help you deliver your baby knows what to do when the time comes. If you are frightened of cancer, arrange for yearly Pap tests and try to understand that the risk is low. If your concern is spreading herpes, realize that the caring and educated person with herpes who is trying to avoid transmitting herpes generally does so with a great deal of success. Find an appropriate person to talk to about herpes, whether that be a health practitioner, or another person with herpes you find at a self-help group, and/or some other knowledgeable and trusted friend.

9. If you believe that your feelings or symptoms fit the category of "clinical depression," you should seek assistance. You should call either your own doctor or a crisis hotline or

go to an emergency room of a hospital. Tell the person there that you are feeling depressed and would like to get some help.

10. Avoid unproven promises of cure. Even if you choose "alternative" methods of therapy, be careful to obtain standard therapy for your medical complaints. Be selective in choosing either a standard or an alternative therapy.

Should I tell my new sexual partner that I have herpes?

This is a very delicate question, and one that no third person outside a relationship can answer. Through my experience talking with people who have herpes, I have heard many opinions expressed. Because of the natural tendency to moralize when dealing with a difficult subject like this, many answers are inadequate. Rather than offer you yet another set of prejudices, I will draw some analogies and ask some questions based upon the concerns of patients as they have expressed them to me. I could pronounce to you the importance of telling your partner as if I were writing you a prescription. Experience tells me, however, that this would be inadequate. Rather, I will present some of the pros and cons for you to consider. When addressing such questions as honesty and integrity, however, please don't look for those answers in a book. For a person making his or her own decision about whether to discuss herpes, past experience, advice from others, and intuition may all be helpful.

We live in an age of informed consent. Recently the courts have decided that the physician must inform the patient about inherent risks from drugs or from surgery. Even if I, as a physician, believe the chances of side effects occurring from a certain drug in any one individual to be very small, I remain duty-bound to discuss them, in order to allow the individual the opportunity to decide. Sharing the information relieves me of the responsibility I would have held had I not explained the side effects. I am still held responsible to uphold my duty to prevent those side effects, if possible. My responsibilities fit the situation, in that I am responsible for my actions, but not responsible for withholding the truth.

As a physician trained to know, or at least expected to know, about side effects, I can easily appreciate that the chances of bad things happening to a particular person are very low. I may choose to avoid discussing all the details, thinking I can avoid creating a needless concern in a patient unlikely to be troubled. I will have saved that patient some anxiety and I will have saved myself having to face an awkward situation which takes time and may be difficult to explain. Indeed, for practical reasons, many physicians do this daily. The physician chooses which side effects to discuss on the basis of their severity and their likelihood of occurrence, as well as on the basis of the individual physician's ease with the patient and how well he or she understands the side effects. Many other factors play a role. For example, how busy is the office? How many times has the same thing been said? How well will the patient understand the information? Will the patient be frightened?

Prior to discussing your herpes with your partner, you have a relationship that closely parallels that of the doctor and the patient. Indeed there may be legal parallels as well. You are holding information in your head about you that may influence how your partner feels or how your partner may act. You have a kind of power over your partner, in the sense that knowledge is power. If you avoid sharing the information, you alter the equal balance in your partnership. Any secret between lovers will change that delicate balance.

On the other hand, your relationship with this person may not be at the stage where you wish to establish that balance or equality. For example, if you are involved in a casual relationship, you may feel that this person is not close enough to share such information with. The risk of transmitting herpes during one encounter in an inactive phase is certainly quite low. Furthermore, any two people in a casual encounter take certain risks in terms of transmitting and receiving infections. If you have a short-term encounter, you generally know that you are taking risks. Nowadays, whether you have herpes or you don't, you are well-advised to avoid casual sexual encounters.

Your decision about whether or not to tell is an individual one. Furthermore, an individual decision may be based upon each situation. It will also be partly based on personal experience. For example, were you told about the risks when you contracted herpes? Could you conceivably have been? Have you previously passed herpes onto anyone? You may decide to withhold the information because it is difficult to tell or because you are a shy or a private person. You may decide to tell because of your conscience or your moral convictions. It may be easier for you to tell than not to tell. It is a matter of personal integrity. Your conscience must compare your right to privacy with your partner's right to informed consent. Choosing to tell is, in some circumstances, the more difficult path to choose. Sometimes it may seem unnecessary. Discussing herpes before having sex may give herpes unwarranted status, especially if you feel in physical control of your infection. Some people note that even though most people have oral herpes, the average person with cold sores does not talk about cold sores before kissing or having oral-genital contact. If a person knows that there is a risk, albeit small, what should be told and what should not be told? Should the person who had one episode of genital herpes five years ago discuss the herpes before each new sexual encounter? If not, where is the line of severity drawn? Should the same individual not discuss oral sores that have recurred monthly since he or she was kissed as a child, because they came from mother and not a lover?

The notion of informed consent implies that the person doing the telling has information to convey. Anything you know about people you are going to make love to may be potentially useful. This is the whole point. If you wish to tell your partner everything, say the following: "By the way, I get recurrences of herpes on my mouth, so when I have a sore we will have to avoid kissing and oral sex," or "By the way, I get recurrences of herpes on my genitals, so when I have a sore we will have to avoid genital sex," or "By the way, I have trouble with my back, so when we sleep together I will need to use a board in the bed," or "By the way, I got sick with salmonella food poisoning back in December and I am now a carrier, so you will have to do the cooking until that is better." Regardless of the situation, you owe it to yourself, your partner, and your relationship to learn the art of discussing herpes.

How should I tell my sexual partner?

There is a lot of advice around, published and unpublished, about herpes discussions. Generally, it is agreed that herpes should be made into no more and no less than it is. Remember that your own overall feeling about this infection will come through in spades when you tell your lover. If you think of yourself in a positive way, that will come through. Avoid preparing for the discussion by painting a picture of impending doom. In other words, stay away from a tone or words that suggest, "Sit down, I have something horrible to tell you," or "Prepare yourself." Your role is simply to inform. Tell your partner everything you know about herpes—what it is, how you know you have it, how you avoid transmitting it, how you have handled telling people before, etc.

Tell your partner early, but not too early. Once you have established mutual trust and realize you want to have a sexual relationship with this person, then talk about herpes *before* you are physically involved. The subject of herpes has a powerful way of curbing spontaneity or spoiling the moment. Thought and sexual arousal are not well-suited partners. *You* must be comfortable with the knowledge you possess since you must serve as an initial resource of information. Despite your other emotions, you must be able to teach with confidence. Avoid using your knowledge to "one-up" or "one-down" the person you are talking with. Instead educate your partner on an equal basis—make it a shared experience.

Expect some expression of fears from your partner. Acceptance without fears could mean your partner knows about herpes already. Alternatively, he or she may not be dealing with the subject. Expressed fears can be dealt with and placed into perspective. Most people will not get up and run from a relationship because of herpes. Remember that herpes is not you, any more than the acne on your back is you or the bump on your nose is you. You need not apologize for having herpes—not to yourself *or* to your partner. You certainly do not need to apologize for talking about it. If you find it especially difficult to talk about herpes in the situation of the casual encounter, you might be advised to opt for avoiding casual relationships, or telling anyway. Going ahead with a casual relationship and avoiding the subject of herpes can be tempting. Entering into a secret situation with a lover, however, is unwise. Nevertheless, this is an individual decision. It all depends upon what is important to you.

What is a self-help group?

Since the dawn of history, people with similar problems and related goals have shared them for mutual benefit. This special kind of community has proven useful for anything from coping with recurring genital sores to fighting world wars. People with herpes may wish to come together for a number of different reasons:

Emotional Support
— participating in group discussions
— sharing similar experiences
— relying on group support
— venting anger in a sympathetic forum
— allaying your own fears by relating them to others
Information Transfer
— making accurate information available to everyone
— keeping abreast of changes in the field
Political Forum
— working with government in deciding key political issues related to herpes, such as education in prevention and treatment and spending of health-care dollars
Charitable Support
— fund raising

— organizing direct monetary support of clinical facilities and herpes hotlines
— supporting basic and clinical research
— training personnel to meet future needs

In deciding how to organize a self-help group, you first need to set goals. Which of the reasons listed above (or not listed above) have brought you together? If emotional support is the only goal, then a local support group is the only necessity. First check to see if a group already exists in your community. You may call local health resource centers, women's health centers, sexually transmitted diseases clinics, public health authorities, or a local herpes clinic, if one exists in your area. Call the national organizations below. They may be able to refer you to a local chapter. It remains critical, in any group, that some or all members be well informed. It would serve no useful purpose if a self-help group were to perpetuate myths and fallacies.

If you want to work for goals on the list other than emotional support, it becomes helpful to join a national organization, if your country has one. People in the United States and Canada can contact:

Herpes Resource Center
P.O. Box 13827
Research Triangle Park, NC 27709
Business telephone: (919) 361-2742

The Herpes Resource Center hotline is open from 9:00 a.m. to 6:00 p.m. Eastern time. The telephone number is (919) 361-2120.

Other important numbers from the resource center's parent organization, the American Social Health Association:
STD National Hotline (U.S.A. only)   (800) 227-8922
National AIDS Hotline (U.S.A. only)   (800) 342-AIDS

What's good about herpes?

The diagnosis of herpes is a crisis. It is an unexpected, uninvited, and unwanted intruder into life. It comes suddenly and strikes in subtle ways. Yet there is always potential in crisis. If nothing else, herpes is a learning experience. Most people who get herpes learn more about biology, medicine, pharmacology, nutrition, and personal communication in the few months following diagnosis than was previously acquired in a lifetime. A herpes crisis is an opportunity to get to know yourself.

Sexual freedom without a care is over. The disadvantages to this are clear—or are they? Herpes adds a new dimension to sex. This has obvious negative potential, but it also promotes honest and open discussion early in relationships. In some cases, openness may upgrade the quality of those relationships. Establishing communication about herpes may make it easier for your partner to discuss serious personal concerns as well. Because of the stress introduced into a personal relationship by herpes, other problems may be brought forward. You would often have had to work through these problems eventually. If your partner picks your herpes as a reason to leave, it may be for the best—as long as it was not based on medical misunderstanding, which can be corrected. In everyone's life at some point, something goes wrong. You might get injured in a car accident or get very sick. Eventually you will die. If this person is going to leave on account of herpes, imagine what would have happened had you been put into a wheelchair or scarred by a fire. Possibly you've found the worm in your apple before you bit too deeply.

Herpes forces people to learn about themselves and about herpes. It forces them to talk about themselves with others. For those who have never been able to talk about intimate feelings and personal matters, herpes can be a springboard.

There is a distinct advantage in knowing definitely that you *have* herpes: unlike the person who has it and does not know, you are relieved of worry about getting it and you are able to distinguish the active herpes phases from the inactive. In fact, the person who knows he or she has herpes and takes care to avoid active phases of infection may be better equipped to avoid transmitting this infection than those who feel they do not have herpes. If you think you don't have herpes, you might be right and you might be wrong.

Herpes is a change. It is a big change for some and a small change for others. The change has some obvious bad points, which must be confronted and dealt with. Changes for the good are also a reality with this infection. Get over the tough parts by facing them directly. Learn the coping methods. Be aware of new developments and, for now, accept the change and the challenge to *normalize* your life in the face of adversity. This virus will probably affect you only once in a while. You have a *virus* for life, but you do not have a *disease* for life. Recurrences may come and go, but herpes will not cause you to lose your job or die a premature or painful death. It may, however, teach you enough in terms of coping that you will continue to grow.

9

SOME SPECIAL PROBLEMS

Homosexuals are really (physiologically) like heterosexuals!
(Catholics are, physiologically, like Protestants; Jews are,
physiologically, like Moslems.) Indeed they are. But the plea for
accepting a minority because it resembles the majority is, in effect,
a denial of the minority's right to be different.

THOMAS SZASZ,
Sex by Prescription

Herpes and the homosexual male

Because of several factors, homosexual men have traditionally
had a much higher risk of contracting sexually transmitted infections than heterosexual men. Changing attitudes because of
AIDS have begun to reduce those risks recently. As we discussed in detail earlier, herpes simplex virus tends to cause infection where it is inoculated. As far as we know, penile sores
in the homosexual are no different from penile sores in the
heterosexual man. However, because anal intercourse may result in inoculation of virus to the anus, herpes may commonly
affect the anus of the homosexual male. *Internal* infection of the
anus is rare in the absence of anal intercourse, although women
commonly experience *external*, or perianal, infection from time
to time.

When the anus is inflamed this is called **proctitis.** Many different infectious agents can cause proctitis, including
gonorrhea, Chlamydia, syphilis, and a host of others. In addition, there are noninfectious causes, such as tearing or abra-

sion from sexual intercourse, ulcerative colitis, etc. Herpes simplex is also a cause for proctitis. Generally speaking (but not always), proctitis results from a primary herpes infection of the rectum. Whereas recurrent herpes in this area tends to be mild and external (in other words, similar to recurrent herpes anywhere else), primary herpes proctitis may result in multiple discomforts during this initial episode. Rectal pain is very common. An urgent feeling of needing to pass stool, whether stool is present or not, is universal. A discharge from the rectum is also common. This discharge may be bloody. Most persons become somewhat constipated and itching may be disturbing. Pains of the low back, buttocks and thigh are often present. Such pains may also accompany genital herpes without proctitis. They are called **sacral paresthesias.** Nearly half of affected men will have difficulty passing urine during this primary episode. Other problems resulting from inflammation of nerves may occur less often, such as temporary impotence. Lesions may be seen externally around the anus or may be present only internally. Fever and swollen glands in the groin are also common. The overwhelming majority of men will have positive virus cultures from the rectum. After one to six weeks the symptoms clear. This infection parallels cervical infection of women in that this primary infection is both internal and external, while recurrent herpes is almost exclusively an external disease.

If I am female and homosexual, can I get herpes?

Yes. There is no reason for you *not* to get genital herpes if you are a lesbian. The risk of acquiring genital herpes may be slightly decreased because of diminished genital-to-genital contact. On the other hand, it will be slightly increased because of increased oral-to-genital contact. Because the main methods of transmission will be oral-to-oral and oral-to-genital, there will be a greater theoretical chance of acquiring herpes simplex virus Type 1. Otherwise, the risks and outcome of a herpes infection are identical in the female homosexual and heterosexual.

Are herpes and AIDS related?

It is not possible to leave the subject of herpes and the homosexual without a comment about **AIDS** or **acquired immune deficiency syndrome.** This disease is not limited to homosexuals, but it has appeared most visibly in this community. Its incidence within high risk categories is doubling every single year, thus qualifying AIDS for the word *epidemic.* Because of infection with a virus called **human immunodeficiency virus,** or **HIV,** persons with AIDS lose certain parts of their immune defense system, specifically the part known as the cellular immune system. These are the lymphocytes spoken about earlier in the book, which, when infected with HIV, eventually die and, therefore, are not available to fight off infection. As a result, persons who develop AIDS may fall victim to any infection or tumor that is generally kept away from our system by these cells. Specifically, tumors such as **Kaposi's sarcoma** or **lymphoma** are found.

Very unusual infections that are not seen in non-immunodeficient people are also encountered, specifically **PCP (Pneumocystis carinii pneumonia),** along with a host of other infections, including herpes simplex. When herpes affects someone with inadequate immunity, many complications can occur. The sores may not heal spontaneously as they normally would; instead they might develop into larger and more extensive ulcers. Parallels exist with the newborn herpes syndrome, where, because of immature immunity, the virus may spread to internal organs. Herpes is highly treatable under these conditions, and intravenous or oral acyclovir (Zovirax®) will generally stop the progression while it is being used. Unfortunately the immune suppression continues. Acyclovir treatment for herpes in the immunosuppressed relieves the problem while the drug is being administered. If the immune suppression continues (as it does in AIDS), herpes infections may recur or progress without continuing therapy.

Herpes has not been, in any way, related to AIDS as a possible cause, although it is a well-known and common complication. The cause of AIDS is now known. HIV seems to spread only by very intimate contact that actually results in an exchange of body fluids between two people. Persons at high risk include intravenous drug users, hemophiliacs (who receive blood products), and homosexual men. Haitian immigrants to the U.S.A. and Canada are also at slightly increased risk not necessarily related to intravenous drugs or homosexuality. Cases with no ethnic, sexual, or habit-related risk factors are also reported, although the risk is exceedingly low if you have no risk factors. Many more people acquire HIV infection compared with the number who will go on to get AIDS. In other words, for most people, even HIV infection is not harmful. For others it leads to a milder illness than AIDS, one which is not fatal. Once again, AIDS has no relationship to herpes, except that people who get AIDS may have difficulty recovering from herpes as well as from a host of other infectious agents.

Can herpes kill?

Yes, herpes can kill. It does so rarely. In general, herpes does not cause serious physical illness in anyone who starts out having regular skin-type herpes, which suddenly, say, goes wild. It can kill only under very specific circumstances: the newborn baby whose immune system has not matured; the adult who, for reasons we do not understand, develops encephalitis, a brain infection; or the person whose immune system fails, resulting in rampant and widespread herpes. In fact, it can generally be said that if you have herpes somewhere on your skin—whether on your lip or your genitals or your toe—herpes is not likely to harm you physically now or in the future.

Will I have herpes for as long as I live?

Yes—and no. As far as we know, once latent infection has been established in the ganglion (which usually occurs before you even realize that you have it the first time), the latent state persists for life. Active infection is not persistent or lifelong, however. As you already know, active phases of infection may sporadically occur depending on whether the herpes reactivates. Some people with a recurrent herpes infection are bothered less frequently after the first couple of years. Others note that their recurrence pattern will just keep going with no change. A high frequency pattern that persists may be quite distressing. This is the person who might look to benefit from drug suppression of outbreaks. Why this persistence of high frequency of outbreaks happens to some individuals is not understood.

For some people with herpes, there comes a time when recurrences cease to be a problem. This burnout of herpes is a pleasant thing if and when it occurs. There are no good explanations for why this happens. Burnout is poorly understood. Possibly the body's immune system has figured out new tricks to kill the virus. If this is the case, scientists have so far been unable to detect any new tricks. Another possibility would be that many of the ganglionic nerve cells affected by latent herpes have now reactivated the virus. Once the infection has reactivated in one cell, that cell probably dies, leaving the person with fewer total affected cells with each recurrence. Nobody knows the actual process. If this burnout phenomenon could be bottled, it would be an excellent patent to hold. It is possible for herpes to seem to slow down for a while and then suddenly get more frequent. In fact, herpes can slow down, speed up, and slow down again. There is no predicting how herpes will behave. If your recurrence pattern becomes more frequent, realize that this will change. It may slow down again, just as it speeded up.

Herpes and eczema

Skin diseases that cause multiple breaks in the integrity of the skin barrier (such as eczema) may, in unusual circumstances, predispose persons with these skin problems to more severe herpes simplex infections. Under these circumstances, during an otherwise uncomfortable, but routine, primary herpes—oral or genital—the virus can work its way into every available skin tear (from eczema) causing skin dissemination. This syndrome is called **eczema herpeticum** or **Kaposi's varicelliform**

eruption. Generally, after about six weeks all lesions heal. Recurrences are not as threatening, since the general immunity of the person is not a problem; the immune problem here seems to be only in the interruption of the normal mechanical skin barrier. Recurrent herpes may wind up in unusual places because of all the sites involved with the primary infection (for example, the scalp area is common).

Persons with significant eczema who develop primary herpes should take extreme care in avoiding self-inoculation. They should also be considered prime candidates for acyclovir, either orally or intravenously, depending upon the severity of the problem.

Occupational herpes hazards: Can I get herpes at work?

The answer depends on the type of work you do. If your contact with people on the job is a potential handshake only, you are at very low risk for contracting herpes at work. If you sell kisses at carnivals, your chances would likely be increased quite a bit. If you sell kisses on the street your chances become close to 100 percent. Many types of other less obvious occupations result in close person-to-person contact. One example occurs at the office of the dentist. The dentist sees many people every day, and he or she has his or her hands in thousands of mouths. The hands are washed very often to prevent the spread of infection. The skin cracks. A patient who has active herpes might donate the virus to a dentist's fingers. The **herpetic whitlow** (Figure 18), or finger infection, is a well-established occupational hazard for the dentist. The dentist unlucky enough to get a herpes on the finger can, in turn, give it to patients by continuing to work without gloves. Dentists (and dental hygienists and dental assistants) with skin rashes or sores on the hands should wear gloves. In fact, I advise new dental students to learn to work with gloves all the time. It is very difficult to relearn the art of dentistry using gloves, but new students who choose to wear gloves with all patients make a wise decision. Recent concerns about hepatitis and AIDS have greatly increased the proportion of dentists wearing gloves.

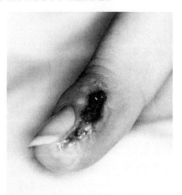

18. Herpetic whitlow. Finger infections with herpes may be caused by Type 1 or Type 2 virus. They might be severe or mild, frequent or infrequent. If tender areas recur on your hand, let your doctor know.

Who else can get a herpetic whitlow? Anyone whose un-gloved hands regularly touch the face or mouth or genitals of another person. Thus, the list includes doctors, nurses, respiratory therapists, wrestlers, and rugby players. In fact, herpes may become a problem in any contact sport. It has been known to occur on many players on an affected team. What happens to the players on that team just before a big challenging event? If you believe in emotional stress as a trigger for herpes, you will then expect that the event will trigger recurrences of sores that peak with virus during the match. These special circumstances have resulted in special names: **herpes gladiatorum** (wrestling), **herpes rugbeiforum** (rugby), etc.

If your occupation has you sitting at a desk, standing at a teller's window, or working in the fields, herpes is not an occupational hazard. If you sit in the diagnostic virus lab as a technician or work as a dental hygienist, the situation is quite different. Remember the cardinal rule. Herpes does not fly through the air with the greatest of ease. It will not jump out at you from the plant in the corner, or from the people sitting to your left, right and behind who have genital herpes and share your toilet seat. However, if you commonly make direct skin-to-skin contact with others, and if the contact might include an area of active herpes on the body, then the possibility of transmission is real. Add a little heat, broken skin, and moisture, as in a wrestling match or a dentist's chair, and you've got a good situation for transmission.

10

NON-GENITAL HERPES INFECTIONS

*So went Satan forth from the presence of the Lord, and smote Job
with sore boils from the sole of his foot unto his crown.*
JOB 2:7

Herpes of the face, mouth, and lips

The lip is the most common location for a herpes simplex infection of any kind. There are probably three to five times as many people with cold sores of the lip than there are people with genital herpes. It is a very common thing to see a facial herpes outbreak. Look at the beach on the first day of bright sunshine. Look at the skiers on the slopes on the first day of snow. The sun triggers the recurrence of a fever blister. Its most common location is the "vermilion border"—the border between the skin of the face and the thinner, pinker mucous membrane of the lips and mouth (See Figure 19).

The fever blister is the recurrent form of herpes of the face. It may erupt repeatedly. Facial sores behave in a similar way to genital sores. They have the same pattern of recurrences, which may be frequent or nonexistent and which are likely to decrease in frequency with time. Facial sores have active phases of infection with similar warnings (prodrome) followed by sores. Because the skin around the lip is a bit drier than the

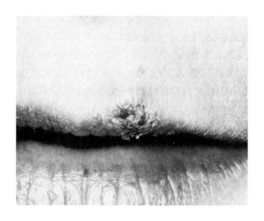

19. A recurrence of oral herpes simplex (herpes labialis). Oral or facial herpes is also commonly found at the tip of the nostrils and around the nose or elsewhere on the face. Instead of recurring by reactivation of herpes simplex from the sacral ganglion, facial herpes recurs from reactivation of virus latent in the trigeminal ganglion.

skin of the genitals, the vesicle (blister) stage is more common.

The classical tale of transmission of oral-facial herpes is as follows: an adult (father, mother, grandmother, aunt, uncle, etc.) transmits herpes to a child as the result of a kiss. However, facial infection could come from any oral-to-oral contact, whether during childhood or adulthood. However, herpes simplex virus does not care where it is inoculated, just as long as it gets inoculated. Thus, oral herpes resulting from genital-to-oral contact is becoming more common.

Like primary herpes infection anywhere, primary facial herpes is usually more severe than recurrent facial herpes. The primary event causes a bigger and more painful collection of skin sores. It also can create a sore throat from sores at the back of the throat. Severe first time mouth infection in a child commonly results in something called **gingivostomatitis.** In this situation almost everything inside the mouth becomes a target for the virus. Ulcers burst out everywhere in the mouth. They may make swallowing food very difficult. Lymph nodes (glands) in the neck may also be swollen and tender. For the usual primary period of two to three weeks, this person is miserable. It may be necessary to use topical anesthetics like lidocaine (Xylocaine®) to help swallowing. Children who suck their thumbs need to stop this habit immediately when they have this infection, in order to avoid painful autoinoculation to the fingers (herpetic whitlow).

Just as with herpes in other parts, the primary or first infection on the face may pass unnoticed. If the child has gingivostomatitis, generally it will be easily diagnosed. If the child has only a sore throat or only a little fever, the whole event may pass unnoticed until the first recurrence. Then the cold sore or fever blister raises its little vesicles on the face. The virus usually reactivates near the lip, but the nose, the cheeks, and even the earlobe are fair game. There are rules for oral herpes like those for genital herpes:

1. Oral herpes is active during active phases. During those phases avoid kissing, especially newborn babies. Also avoid oral sex, thumb sucking, nose picking, and eye rubbing.
2. Keep contact lenses out of your mouth at all times, especially when cold sores are active.
3. Stay away from your dentist when you have a cold sore. It would not be nice for the dentist.
4. What about treatment? Many of the same rules apply here as for genital herpes, so they will not be repeated. Oral acyclovir offers only minor benefits for recurrent oral-labial herpes and is generally not prescribed in this setting. Acyclovir ointment, idoxuridine drops, and ara-A ointment are not beneficial for this problem and are best avoided. You should also avoid a host of other drugs being sold outside of the drugstore. They are listed in the treatment section for reference.
5. A wet warm face cloth is used to soak the affected area. Then blow dry with a hair dryer set on low. This will soothe the area. Ice, ether, alcohol, BHT, soap, and vaseline treatments are best avoided.

Herpes of the eye

Herpes of the eye is very much like herpes elsewhere. There is often a primary first episode with pain and swelling. Primary infections may be followed by recurrences. As for all herpes infections, recurrences cause less systemic (total body) involvement and less tissue is upset, etc. However, recurrences in the eye may lead to local complications, which can potentially interfere with vision. If these progress, and/or if the complications become quite severe, decreased vision in the infected eye can result.

Generally, herpes of the eye is caused by herpes simplex Type 1. The time of infection and source of virus are identical to oral herpes. In other words, a baby or young child, more often than a young adult, may become infected with herpes simplex, generally resulting from mouth contact with someone close, for example, a kiss from Mom or Dad. The person doing the kissing may or may not have a recognizable fever blister. The most ironic situation arises when a small child falls and scrapes the face or forehead near the eye. Mom, wishing to soothe the pain, kisses it to make it better. The result? Herpes has ready-made access to epithelial cells from the cut. The inoculation comes from the kiss. As far as the virus is concerned, this was as easy as using a needle for access. There are no barriers to jump across. Direct inoculation to the eye, specifically, is also made easy because the barrier is generally so thin. The protective layer of the eye is not tough and thick like skin, but rather thin and fragile. Transmission from genital sores on one person to the eye of another through direct contact of genitals to eye is possible, but it is not commonly seen.

Primary herpes of the eye

Once inoculated, an infection may occur some 2 to 21 days later. The primary, or first, event with ocular (eye) herpes is characteristic yet sometimes difficult to diagnose. Generally (not always), only one eye is affected. Redness and discomfort of the eye develops. This is the appearance of pinkeye or **conjunctivitis.** The sac protecting the eye is inflamed. When you pull down the bag under your eye and stare into the mirror, you are looking at the membrane called the conjunctiva. Conjunctivitis is an extremely common infection in children. Most times the virus causing this is not herpes simplex. A very common cause of conjunctivitis in children, for instance, is **adenovirus,** which commonly occurs in small epidemics or outbreaks from swimming pools, schools, and so forth. Unlike herpes simplex, adenovirus is a very hearty virus, capable of withstanding drying. It does "fly through the air with the greatest of ease." Adenovirus usually involves both eyes. Other viruses, bacteria, and Chlamydia can also cause conjunctivitis. Along with the red, uncomfortable eye comes a watery, tearing discharge. Often the neck glands are swollen. In this case, a lymph node (gland) just to the front of the ear on the same side as the eye infection is inflamed and tender. The eyelid may be swollen on the involved side. Often (but not always) a careful search for typical herpes lesions (see pictures in Chapter 3) will yield a positive result. They may be on the eyelid, under the eyelashes, or even on the forehead, in the hair, near the nose, or near the mouth.

At this point, all is well in terms of vision. The person may feel sick, but vision is normal. The whole process of conjunctivitis lasts about two or three weeks. The physician may elect to send you to an eye specialist (ophthalmologist), who may use antiviral (antiherpes) eye drops. There is no information proving that treatment at this point is effective or even helpful in preventing more severe eye involvement. Despite that, if it were my eye, I'd put in the drops.

Usually herpes conjunctivitis just heals at that stage and that's it. Primary herpes may occasionally affect the cornea, however. If this occurs, the person will notice that the symptoms described for conjunctivitis are just beginning to clear when new, quite different, symptoms begin. During herpes conjunctivitis there may have been swelling and inflammation, but vision was not affected. As **keratitis** begins, however, vision may blur. Keratitis is a name for inflammation of the cornea. Blurred vision resulting from herpes means the cornea is inflamed. The cornea covers the front of the eye where light first enters. It is a protective outer coat of transparent material. Keratitis is a much more serious problem than conjunctivitis, since the conjunctiva is a protective membrane which we don't actually look through. As shown in Figure 20, however, we look through the cornea. It is the part just under a contact lens. Inflammation of the cornea leads to blurred vision. If a deep opaque scar of the cornea were to develop, decreased vision in the involved eye might result. Universally, with keratitis, the eye feels gritty to its owner, as if it had a sandpaper surface, and it responds to bright light with a spasm of pain called **photophobia.**

If you suspect keratitis, go to an eye specialist or **ophthalmologist.** The tests to make the diagnosis of keratitis can only

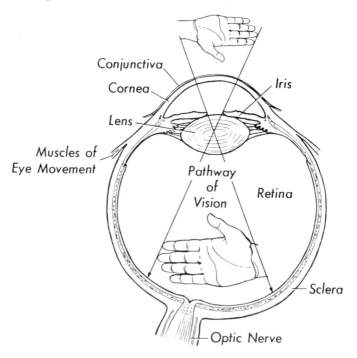

20. *The anatomy of the eye. The conjunctiva, which forms a protective outer sac around the front of the eye (sort of like "eye skin"), is the first place for herpes of the eye to affect. Recurrences can be a problem because of involvement of the cornea, since the cornea is part of the visual pathway. If the cornea is blurred, it may have the effect of blurring the vision. If only the conjunctiva is affected, vision is not blurred.*

be done properly by someone with the right equipment and experience in eye diseases. In order to see the lesion properly, the specialist will need a slit lamp, which is a sort of rotating microscope that allows the doctor to see an enlarged view of your eye as you hold your head still on a resting post. A dye called rose bengal or fluorescein will be used, making a herpes sore stand out clearly. The diagnosis of herpes depends mostly on the specialist's opinion, although he or she may also wish to do a virus test at the same time, like those described earlier in the book.

If herpes simplex is confirmed, you (or your child) may be treated with several things:

1. An **antiviral agent.** There are several good antiherpes drugs that can be used in the eye. Locally applied drugs help a lot in the eye, often a very different situation from herpes elsewhere. Useful drugs for the eye include idoxuridine (IDU, Stoxil®, Herplex®), adenine arabinoside (ara-A, Vira-A®), and trifluorothymidine (TFT, Viroptic®, Trifluridine). A host of other chemicals are also being developed for use here. It is very arguable which drug should be used first or next and why. Stick with your physician's decision.
2. A **cycloplegic.** This is a drug which relaxes a muscle in the eye called the ciliary muscle. It will cause your eye to dilate and relax just as it does when you get drops at the eye doctor's office. This reduces the pain of photophobia.
3. **Pain relievers** are generally useful here, and these will vary depending on the need and the individuals involved.
4. **Sunglasses** or very dark glasses may also help.
5. Early keratitis is often treated with **debridement.** This is a minor surgical cleaning procedure and is quite helpful for early keratitis. It is not used in later stages of keratitis.

Recurrent herpes of the eye

We have seen that primary herpes of the eye generally causes only a self-limited two or three week period of conjunctivitis and does not affect vision. Furthermore, we have reviewed what happens to a few people as the conjunctivitis improves; that is, they get keratitis, which can cause further problems. When ocular herpes recurs, it does so by causing recurrent keratitis. Eventually, the feeling of grittiness and pain may decrease because herpes of the eye causes a loss of feeling of the eye surface (cornea) called **hypoesthesia.** Instead there may be a recurrence of a feeling of irritation that something like sand or dust is in the eye. With each recurrence there may be an increase in tearing. There may be a recurrence of eye pain on exposure to light (photophobia). There may also be a simultaneous occurrence of sores on the lips, face, mouth, or nose. The eye specialist will assess you each time this occurs to make sure it is herpes once again.

You may be treated with the same drugs listed for primary herpes of the eye. Drops of cortisone or any of its derivatives, which are *absolutely contraindicated* during conjunctivitis and early keratitis, *may* become useful when carefully administered during some deeper forms of keratitis called **disciform keratitis** or **stromal keratitis.** (An incomplete list of cortisone drops includes Betnesol®, Cortisporin®, Decadron®, Metimyd®, Metreton®[1], Neo-Cortef®[1], Neo-Medrol®[1], Optimyd®[1], and Sofracort®[1].) Generally, cortisone drops are combined with a specific antiviral drug so that the virus growth is held back. The eye specialist may wish to repeatedly perform minor surgical scraping procedures, called **debridement.**

Herpes encephalitis

Encephalitis means inflammation of the brain tissue. It is different from **meningitis** which means inflammation of the protective sac around the brain called the **meninges.** In some clinical situations both brain tissue and meninges become infected at the same time with the same agent and this would be

---

[1]These drops contain mixtures of antibiotics and cortisone derivatives. Mixtures are generally not useful for herpes at any stage. Avoid any from this list during the early stages of herpes.

called **meningoencephalitis.** Herpes simplex can cause either encephalitis or meningitis. The outcome is very different.

Herpes encephalitis in an adult is a very serious disease. Without treatment, encephalitis is often deadly. With treatment it may be deadly also, or it may cause significant brain damage. It does not have any correlation, whatsoever, to herpes of the mucous membrane, skin, or eyes. It is a disease of its own, which happens for reasons we do not understand. A person with genital herpes is neither prone to, nor protected from, herpes encephalitis.

Herpes meningitis, on the other hand, is a direct complication of genital or anal herpes. Meningitis should not be confused with encephalitis. It commonly occurs as a symptom of primary herpes. It may cause a severe headache. It may cause eye pain when looking at light (photophobia). It does not cause permanent damage to the nervous system. Left alone, meningitis gets better and almost never recurs. Treated, it also gets better and almost never recurs.

Herpes encephalitis may also occur during neonatal herpes. The neonatal herpes symptoms and its prevention are discussed in Chapter 6. Remember that neonatal herpes encephalitis usually, but not always, follows genital herpes in the mother. Most mothers giving birth to babies with this problem never thought they had herpes. We need to find these people because studies are showing that we can prevent neonatal herpes quite effectively by doing a cesarean section during active herpes. The diagnosis must be known, however, in order to take preventative action.

Herpes encephalitis of the adult occurs by an altogether different mechanism. For some reason, which we do not understand, herpes simplex makes its way to the brain. It may get there by any number of ways. It most likely gets to the brain by traveling up a nerve called the trigeminal nerve. Normally, herpes of the face, lip, nose, or eye stops at the trigeminal ganglion where it stays as a latent infection (see Chapter 2). In the rare case of encephalitis, however, the virus does not stop for a latency rest at the ganglion. Instead, it keeps traveling right to the brain tissue. This syndrome is rare and is seen both in people who get facial herpes and in people who do not. Once inside the brain, herpes picks a spot for infection. That spot can be, literally, anywhere. However, it is most commonly in an area of the brain called the **temporal lobe,** more or less underneath the temple or the ear. Oddly enough, the virus stays right there and just damages the area of the lobe it is in. In so doing, however, it causes swelling and inflammation. This can result in more widespread damage, because the brain is encased in a cranial vault of bone with no room for swelling.

Herpes encephalitis occurs at any age from infancy to old age. Common complaints in adults or older children include fever, which is present in 90 percent of cases. A change in consciousness (something ranging from sleepiness or disoriention to deep coma) is nearly universal. The patient may complain early in the course of infection of headache. Commonly, there is a sudden personality change or bizarre behavior. A seizure (fit, convulsion) may occur. Speech may be abnormal. Paralysis or weakness on one side of the body may sometimes occur. In most cases paralysis like this results not from herpes but from stroke.

It is difficult to diagnose herpes encephalitis. Several tests may be performed in the search for the answer, among them **electroencephalography** (EEG), **computerized tomography** (CT scan), and a **brain scan.** None of these tests, unfortunately, is specific. As with all herpes infections, the diagnosis depends upon finding the virus. In the case of herpes encephalitis, the herpes simplex virus is in brain tissue and only brain tissue. Thus, the diagnosis is made by brain biopsy. This is an operative procedure, requiring a neurosurgeon who drills a small hole in the skull and removes a small piece of brain tissue for examination. The biopsy itself carries minimal danger when compared to leaving infection of this severity untreated or wrongly treated. Experts agree that if this diagnosis is considered, a brain biopsy should be performed.

Treatment for herpes encephalitis is intravenous acyclovir (Zovirax®). This drug is quite helpful in decreasing an otherwise 75 percent death rate. It is not a miraculous therapy for everyone, because damage may have been done to vital brain tissue before therapy has had the chance to work. Unfortunately, until we can make this diagnosis earlier,[2] we will be stuck with a frightening and serious disease, which is very uncommon in the adult and which has no connection whatsoever to genital herpes.

[2]Making an early diagnosis in herpes encephalitis is truly an important and exciting challenge for the future. Scientists have tried blood tests, spinal fluid tests, and scans. In order to make the diagnosis earlier, we are going to have to devise a "noninvasive test"—one which does not "invade" the body as a brain biopsy does. Recently it has been suggested that one of the thymidine analog drugs or other drugs that are specifically included by virus-infected cells and excluded by healthy cells might be labelled with a radioactive tag. Then, if herpes encephalitis is suspected, the drug would be given by vein. A special camera that detects the radioactive label might take a picture of the herpes from outside the body! This trick may work, but it has only been tried in animals, which get very different kinds of encephalitis. It will be vital to watch this very carefully in the future. It may be that herpes encephalitis is not rare at all, but that it is only rarely so severe that a brain biopsy must be performed (resulting in a diagnosis of herpes encephalitis). After all, not too many physicians do a brain biopsy on every person with a headache or a personality change! Imagine if herpes were the cause of schizophrenia and it became treatable with an antiviral drug!

11

THERAPY NOW AND LATER

For every evil under the sun
There is a remedy or there is none
If there be one, seek till you find it
If there be none, never mind it.
MOTHER GOOSE

Accepted therapy today: What can I do right now?

If you have *primary* genital herpes or think you might have:

1. Go to your doctor or clinic. Have a trained professional diagnose the problem and confirm the presence of herpes by a virus test (culture test or fluorescence test or electron microscope test).
2. A blood test for syphilis should be done and it should be repeated in a couple of weeks.
3. If the pain is severe, you may wish to discuss obtaining a pain reliever by prescription to help you "make it through the nights."
4. Take a very warm shower in order to run warm water over the area three to four times a day. Occasionally an individual finds water on these sores to be absolutely intolerable. If that happens to you, stop using water. Most people find water to be very helpful, however.
5. When you get out of the shower or bath, blow the genital

148

area dry with a hair dryer with adjustable temperatures. Set it on low or cool, being careful not to burn yourself.

6. Make sure you are passing urine without difficulty. If you try to go and it won't come, try again. Try urinating in the shower or tub to decrease the sting. Turn on the sink tap for background noise. Outside of the bath, you might try to direct the urine stream away from your sores with a bit of rolled up toilet tissue. Pouring warm water over the area using a glass of water may also be helpful. Some people have found that drinking a lot of water (eight glasses a day) dilutes the urine enough that it hurts less. Others point out that this increases the number of times you have to urinate. Whether you would rather it hurt more intensely on fewer occasions or less intensely on more occasions is up to you.

7. If you cannot pass urine and you've tried several times, wait a couple of hours—even three or four. If there is still no result, you must have medical attention. Not passing urine can lead to serious problems, which are totally preventable. If you can find your own doctor, call or visit him or her. If the physician is difficult to locate, go to the emergency room of a local hospital.

8. Avoid tight undergarments. If possible, avoid undergarments altogether. Try loose fitting things, made of pure cotton. If you are able to go to work, upon returning home, take off your clothes and take a shower, or soak in the tub. Leave your clothes off if you can.

9. You *should* be treated with a drug called acyclovir (Zovirax®). Generally, it should be given orally as soon as the diagnosis of a first episode of genital herpes is suspected. Treatment is continued for at least 10 days, or longer if the lesions are not healed by then. A topical (ointment) preparation is also available but it is less effective than the preferred oral form. If hospitalization is necessary, this agent can be given intravenously. Drugs other than acyclovir are being tested. For now, all others are in the experimental stages or are unproven. You may wish to receive oral acyclovir or be hospitalized for intravenous treatment. If your outbreak is quite severe and giving you

trouble walking, or if your head feels like the top is going to come off, or if you are having trouble urinating, then intravenous acyclovir may be the best route. More information on acyclovir is available later in this chapter.

10. Avoid because they may be worse than doing nothing:
   — cortisone cream or ointment
   — antibiotic cream or ointment
   — any cream or ointment unless it contains a useful, specific antiherpes drug
   — vaseline
   — antibiotics (unless you have a clear-cut secondary infection)
   — alcohol (just because it stings)
   — ether (because it stings and can catch fire)
   — DMSO (dimethyl sulfoxide)

   Avoid because they are of no proven benefit:
   — L-lysine
   — BHT
   — idoxuridine (IDU, Stoxil®, Herplex-D®)

11. If you are pregnant during primary herpes, let your physician know and read Chapter 6 of this book. Take care of yourself by giving yourself time to heal, treating other infections if they are present, and treating your herpes.

12. Remember that it is hard to learn and figure out everything all at once. The answers will come. The ability to cope will also come. There is no truth to the rumors that stress will make your primary herpes worse. It is very distressing to have primary herpes. Accept the stress for now. Follow the suggestions above to take care of the immediate problem.

After my primary herpes is over

At this point, it is usually not clear whether you will have recurrences. Generally, most people with Type 2 herpes will get some recurrences. Type 1 may also recur, although less frequently than Type 2, in general. If you don't get recurrences, you do not need treatment. Treatment would be truly unwise unless there is something to treat. Latent infection inside the ganglion does not hurt you. By itself, latent infection is untreatable by anything available in the drug department. Leave latent infection alone. Some will have you believe that you can intervene and affect this latent infection with a drug. For now, you cannot.

What if I am having recurrent herpes, or think I might have it?

You should learn about active phases of infection so you can avoid sore-to-skin contact when necessary (see Chapter 3).

You may wish to use the hot showers and hair dryer routine described for primary herpes, depending upon the amount of discomfort your sores cause when they are active.

You may decide to try therapy, or you may decide not to. If your recurrences are mild and only come every four or five months, or less often, you would probably be best advised to leave well enough alone.

The average recurrence of herpes lasts about six to ten days from start to finish. Topical acyclovir (Zovirax®) ointment is not helpful enough in recurrent herpes to be considered worthwhile. In some studies it killed the herpes virus a little faster during recurrences than if it had not been used. Concerning topical acyclovir, Dr. Richard Reichman and his coworkers reported the following results of a carefully conducted trial in the *Journal of Infectious Diseases:* "There were no significant differences between the [topical] acyclovir and placebo-treated groups of either sex in time to crusting of lesions, time required for lesions to heal, time to cessation of pain, or in frequency with which new lesions developed during their course of therapy. Mild, transient burning or pain associated with application of the study medication was a common complaint." When it comes down to the nitty-gritty of getting rid of the lesions, topical acyclovir is not good enough to bother with. In fact, even using topical acyclovir (Zovirax®) for recurrent herpes by starting it very early, at home with the first sign of recurrence (prodrome), has no useful clinical effect. It should be avoided for recurrent herpes, altogether, in my opinion.

The oral form of acyclovir is now available on prescription from your doctor. Unlike the ointment, acyclovir by mouth has been shown to speed the time to healing of recurrences. It can also decrease the rate of very frequent recurrences. Oral use of this agent is discussed in detail later in this chapter.

Several other forms of newer treatments are being developed and are in varying stages of testing (see pages 172–191).

The following compounds have been rigorously tested in scientific studies and have been shown to be **ineffective.** The ones which are marked (*) are also considered worse than using nothing, either because they may prolong lesions or complications, or because of real or potential harmful effects or local discomfort upon application:

— alcohol applied to the sores
— Bacille Calmette-Guerin (BCG) vaccine*
— chloroform* applied to the sores
— DMSO* (dimethyl sulfoxide, Rimso-50®) applied to the sores
— ether* applied to the sores
— idoxuridine (IDU, Stoxil®, Herplex-D®) applied to the sores
— levamisole*
— ointments or creams not containing a specific antiherpes drug (including cortisone, antibiotics, etc.)*
— oral polio vaccine
— photodynamic inactivation (light and red dye treatments)*
— smallpox vaccine*
— topical acyclovir (Zovirax®)
— topical adenine arabinoside (Vira-A®, ara-A)

A new era of treatment for herpes began with the licensing of oral acyclovir: Make up your own mind

In December of 1977, a biochemist by the name of Dr. Gertrude Elion and a chemist by the name of Dr. Howard Schaeffer, along with four coworkers, communicated their discovery of a new chemical compound to the world. Its molecular formula is $C_8H_{11}N_5O_3$. These scientists from Wellcome Research Laboratories called their compound by its chemical name 9-(2-hydroxyethoxymethyl) guanine. Back then, the chemical also went by its code name, BW248U, or its descriptive name, acycloguanosine. This was modified to the official generic term "acyclovir" which now carries the trade name, Zovirax®.

Fewer than eight years later, acyclovir was released in oral form for use by people with genital herpes infections. The year 1985 marked the beginning of a new era of therapy for genital herpes. Until then, home remedies had been the rule of the day. Dietary supplements and food additives were used along with a host of other treatments (most often unsuccessfully) in an attempt to change the frequency of recurrences. The story is different with acyclovir, however. It has now been proven beyond the shadow of a doubt that oral acyclovir does the following:

1. Taken for five days, beginning at the outset of one recurrence of genital herpes, acyclovir shortens that episode.
2. Taken every single day, in doses ranging from two to five tablets or capsules per day, acyclovir can prevent most outbreaks. It reduces the severity of the others which "break through."
3. Taken during first episodes of genital herpes, acyclovir shortens the episode by one week on average. It lessens the severity of urinary discomfort and swollen lymph nodes.

These are dramatic clinical findings, which will make a big difference to many people who have problems with their herpes infections. Yet despite the exciting findings surrounding this agent, it is not for everyone. For those who need it, oral acyclovir can be a very effective treatment. But knowing who needs it can be very difficult.

This section outlines the way in which this drug works, along with its effects on the virus and the human body—the information you'll need to know when deciding with your physician whether you want to try it. As always, it is in that setting—with your own physician—that both of you must decide on a course of action for you, personally. This section is just for information, in order to present a balanced approach. The doses and indications for use are not necessarily those described in the official drug inserts. Therefore, *any decision regarding use of this drug should be made with your own physician,* who will take these other factors into account.

MECHANISM OF ACTION

Acyclovir is called a **nucleoside analog.** Although chemically altered, acyclovir is a "spitting image" of a real nucleoside. In many biological ways it can behave just like a real nucleoside. Actually there are four *real* nucleosides that are used by the cells in our bodies to make DNA. DNA is also called the double helix, which describes its shape. It is the hereditary material— the code transmitted from parent to child. It determines who you are, from the shape of your nose to the color of your skin. In fact, every cell in every part of the human body contains DNA. In many of these cells, DNA is rapidly dividing in order to create new cells from the old. Even though we may have stopped growing in overall size, many of our cells need constant replacing, such as sperm-making cells, or white blood cells which fight off infection. Stomach and intestinal cells are also continuously being sloughed off as dead, then digested and replaced with brand new cells containing new DNA. In fact, even if one never has children, one is being constantly reproduced in small bits throughout life. These cellular reproductive processes all require healthy, intact DNA as the basic code for the continuation of the system.

This double-stranded DNA is the same basic type of coding system used by herpes simplex virus. The "parent" virus literally passes on its code to its "offspring" by giving it copies of its DNA. Once the new virus possesses the code, a bit of nutrient is all that is required to make a whole new virus copy. In other words, once the DNA "template" (like a plaster mold) is in place, the reproductive process can carry on.

These four nucleosides are the parts used to make up the

DNA code. Depending upon the nucleoside sequence, these nucleosides will determine the size of your nose (if they are part of your DNA), or the size of your skin sore (if they come from your herpes virus). DNA looks much like a ladder as it grows. One side of the ladder is used as the "template" (mold), which is made up of a certain sequential code. Let's say for the purpose of discussion that this code has the following sequence: AGCTCAC. This is seen on the left in Figure 21, labeled template, read from bottom to top. According to the rules of DNA growth and reproduction, there is an exact system for connecting nucleosides, which cannot be altered.

The first rule of the system says that A's always get linked

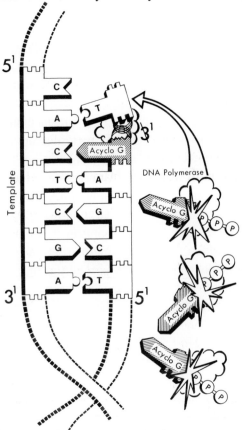

21. *A new strand of DNA is being made on the right to complement the "template" strand on the left. The sequence has to fit perfectly, but once acyclovir is inserted new nucleosides cannot enter. This terminates the DNA chain.*

side by side to T's; G's always get linked to C's. Tracing the growth of the DNA ladder depicted in the figure, then, the first rung pairs A to T, then G to C, then C to G, then T to A. Each nucleoside has a unique shape for linking only with its complementary nucleoside. The new strand is built in parallel to its complementary mold—the template strand.

The second rule of this strict system says that the new strand grows in the 3′ (pronounced "three prime") direction by tightly interlocking with the last nucleoside in the chain. Chemically, this second rule assures that 5′ ends link up to 3′ ends so that everything stays oriented with the precision of a military march. The 5′ to 3′ linkup is orchestrated by the system catalyst, which goes by the name DNA polymerase. DNA polymerase makes sure that the last 3′ end finds the next nucleoside in exactly the right orientation so that it hooks tightly to the 5′ end of the next nucleoside, which then exactly complements the opposing nucleoside in the template—and so on, and so on, and so on.

Acyclovir does not possess a 3′ end. In most other ways, however, acyclovir resembles the G in the linkup system. In fact, originally this was called "acycloguanosine" or "acyclo G" as it is depicted in the figure. DNA polymerase picks up this acyclo G thinking it is a real G and sucessfully links its 5′ end up to the 3′ end of the growing strand. Following the rules, of course, G is across from C. Continuing in its unyielding and single-minded fashion, DNA polymerase grabs up a new nucleoside component for the next part of the link in this assembly line of life. In our figure, this is a T brought in to pair up with an A in the template. It takes the 5′ end of T and tries to link it up with the 3′ end of G. But acyclo G has no 3′ end, so no linkup is possible. This results in termination of the DNA chain. It stops the growth of the DNA chain as a key broken inside of a lock prevents another key from opening the door.

In addition, acyclovir is able to play a double jeopardy scene. Not only does it terminate the chain, but it inhibits the very enzyme that placed it there—DNA polymerase. DNA polymerase is the chain growth catalyst—in the metaphor sense, this enzyme is the robot that brings the nucleoside pieces together to link them according to the rules. In other words, not only does it ruin the new DNA chain while it is being formed, but it attacks the robot responsible for attaching the links. This is graphically depicted by little explosions to the right of the chain. To DNA, then, acyclovir is a deadly poison. As far as we know, in the test tube, acyclovir can interfere with both human DNA growth and viral DNA growth. So why is this drug not a poison to humans? The answer requires one more short biochemistry lesson.

Nucleosides do not actually make up the rungs of the ladder of DNA. Actually, before they can be used for making DNA, these nucleosides must first be converted to nucleotides. This means they obtain three phosphates inside the cell, designated Ⓟ in the drawing. Special enzymes enhance this transformation (or activation) with phosphate groups. The activation steps pave the way for insertion of these chemicals into DNA. Without their phosphates these nucleosides just sit there. Once activated by three phosphates, however, these chemicals, now called nucleotides, make up the DNA sequence.

Acyclovir, being a nucleoside analog, also just sits there until activated to acyclovir -Ⓟ-Ⓟ-Ⓟ, also called acyclovir triphosphate. Acyclovir -Ⓟ-Ⓟ-Ⓟ is the nucleotide and is a deadly poison to any DNA it finds—yours, mine, or herpes.

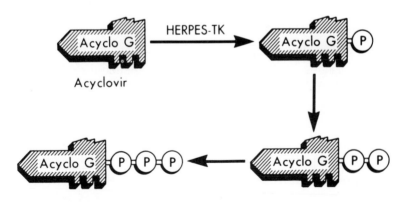

22. *Acyclovir is activated by the herpes enzyme called thymidine kinase. In its activated, or phosphorylated, form it can be further changed to acyclovir triphosphate. Only the triphosphate accomplishes the DNA killing as pictured in Figure 21.*

Happily, acyclovir does not even get its first Ⓟ until it comes across an enzyme called thymidine kinase. Thymidine kinase, or TK, obtains the Ⓟ for acyclovir and attaches it. This starts the ball rolling toward attachment of the series of three Ⓟ's, and drug activation has begun. Luckily, the virus makes lots of this TK. Our own cells don't make much, and what they do make does not readily accomplish this activation step. In fact, scientists from Burroughs Wellcome have shown that herpes-infected cells will add this Ⓟ group as much as 120 times faster than our own healthy cells. There is little doubt that the ability of herpes TK to activate acyclovir accounts for this drug's potency in killing cells infected with this virus, while leaving normal, healthy cells largely unaffected. This special activation by herpes is depicted in Figure 22.

In summary, acyclovir-Ⓟ-Ⓟ-Ⓟ is the "real" drug and it is only made in high quantity in cells with herpes infection. Herpes-infected cells are the only ones that are immediately affected by this DNA poison, which stops the production of virus inside of the cell. Acyclovir-Ⓟ-Ⓟ-Ⓟ is made mainly and most quickly in virus-infected cells; however, it is not made *exclusively* in virus-infected cells. Normal human cells *will* phosphorylate acyclovir although only at very, very low levels—almost below our ability to detect the chemical, but not quite.

POSITIVE EFFECTS OF ORAL ACYCLOVIR

First episodes

First episodes of genital herpes have been effectively treated with oral acyclovir. Dr. Yvonne Bryson from UCLA found first episodes to be shortened by 3.0 days in men and 4.2 days in women. In the more severe (primary) episodes the time was decreased by 9.0 days in men and 6.2 days in women. The duration of virus shedding (positive cultures) was also reduced. When more severe symptoms were present, the positive effects from acyclovir were also seen as reductions in pain, lymph node discomfort, urinary discomfort, and general body aches; these symptoms started to improve by day three or four in most people taking acyclovir.

Dr. Mertz and coworkers from many centers across the United States and Canada reported a reduction of five days in men and two days in women with full-blown primary infections. This was, statistically speaking, of borderline significance for women. Among patients with nonprimary first episodes of genital herpes, the median time to healing was reduced by four days by acyclovir, but this reduction was also not statistically significant. Nevertheless, a dramatic reduction in formation of new lesions (18 percent vs. 62 percent) was seen and this difference was highly significant. In the same fashion as Dr. Bryson's study, Dr. Mertz showed the duration of virus shedding was reduced in patients receiving oral acyclovir when compared to those receiving placebo (look-alike sugar pills).

Dr. Bryson has now followed the patients from this original study for several years after. She recently reported that the true primary patients (see Chapter 3) who received acyclovir during this study are now having significantly fewer episodes of recurrences after the first year of infection. Other investigators have not found this, but they have also not looked beyond the first year. If this holds up in future studies, it would be further evidence to support the importance of using oral (or intravenous) acyclovir during the primary infection.

In summary, oral acyclovir works minor wonders in severe first episodes of herpes. It makes people feel better faster, although several days are still required for healing, especially during severe primary episodes. Because of this drug's positive effect on urine problems, which can occur commonly in first episodes, it is especially worthy of consideration by people with urinary complaints or those having marked discomfort. Because of the reduction in new lesion formation, which might not be apparent right at the beginning of an episode, oral acyclovir should be used in all patients with first episodes of genital herpes as soon as the diagnosis is suspected, unless the episode is very mild *and* nearly healed when first seen.

Recurrences

Dr. Richard Reichman from the University of Vermont, along

with investigators from San Diego, Seattle, Edmonton, and Montreal, has reported findings on 250 patients with recurrent genital herpes. The drug was administered as 200 mg five times per day for five days. In comparison to placebo, acyclovir-treated recurrences were shorter by 0.7 days on average, although when patients treated themselves earlier, during their warning signs (like skin tingling or itching), healing times on acyclovir were shorter by 1.0 day (average). Despite shorter times to healing, the duration of the symptoms of recurrences (itching or pain) were not proven to be positively affected by acyclovir treatment. No differences have been noted between drug or placebo.

Prophylaxis

Many investigative groups have analyzed the effects of oral acyclovir in preventing recurrent herpes. All have found essentially the same positive results. Each has a slightly different study design. Dr. Steve Strauss from the National Institutes of Health, along with his coworkers, studied 35 healthy adults with genital herpes. Each participant had a recurrence frequency of greater than one episode per month. On average, the patients treated with acyclovir took 137.7 days to get a recurrence after starting treatment, whereas placebo recipients required about 45 days on average to get a recurrence. After the treatment was stopped, people from both groups got recurrences within a month on average.

The Seattle study reported by Dr. John Douglas and coworkers showed equally impressive results. They divided their groups into low dose (two 200 mg capsules per day) and high dose (five 200 mg capsules per day). Their patients had had six recurrences or more in the year prior to study. Of 47 placebo recipients, 44 (94 percent) had recurrences during four months of therapy. However, only 13 of 45 patients (29 percent) had recurrences on low-dose treatment, and 18 of 51 (35 percent) had recurrences on high-dose treatment. In fact, the recurrences they did have were shorter. After the drug was withdrawn, both groups developed recurrences once again.

From London, England, Dr. Mindel and associates reported

similar findings. Fifty-six patients with at least four episodes per year were given 200 mg four times per day or placebo. The recurrence rate was 1.4 per month in those on placebo and 0.05 per month on acyclovir. Again, no differences were seen after the drug was withdrawn.

Several other studies not listed here have added to this impressive acyclovir record. We recently reported an oral acyclovir prophylaxis trial from Vancouver. For enrollment in this trial, which was performed simultaneously by Dr. Joe Portnoy in Montreal, volunteers had at least one episode per month for one year or more. Each person received three capsules of acyclovir 200 mg or placebo every day for six months, although if a visible lesion developed during the study, that episode was treated for five days with five capsules per day. During the treatment period, approximately one-third of our volunteers receiving acyclovir had no episodes and another one-third had only one episode of visible lesions. The people receiving placebo continued to have their usual—more than one episode per month. During this study, however, we recorded episodes of warning only (tingling or itching but no visible sore develops) and found that they were much more common in the group of acyclovir recipients. In fact, Dr. Strauss reported similar findings in his study. This would suggest the likely possibility that recurrences recycled and began in our study, despite acyclovir prophylaxis. They did so at just about the same rate as without treatment. However, these "beginnings" most often did not develop into visible sores. Nobody knows if these warnings are associated with shedding of virus from skin. After several months of acyclovir suppression, patients usually stop experiencing most of these nonlesional episodes, as if the body finally "realizes" that it is not getting most of its recurrences. Nevertheless, it would be wise to refrain from genital intercourse during these "beginnings," should they occur in you.

Dr. Greg Mertz has reported his findings on a very large study of oral acyclovir, recently completed, where several hundred patients took acyclovir for one and/or two years. The dose was 400 mg twice daily. Acyclovir maintained its suppressive effects over this time. Generally, about 25 percent of patients will break through with one recurrence every three to four months. The safety record of acyclovir over two years remains very good.

Another study of recent vintage shows that one tablet per day is also effective—if (and only if) this tablet is four times the normal dose (800 mg). If and when this tablet is approved for general use, it will make remembering the "daily herpes pill" a bit more convenient.

SIDE EFFECTS

In terms of the short-term side effects of acyclovir, this drug appears to be extremely safe. At the doses used orally for this drug, blood acyclovir levels for up to at least two years are well below the toxic range. Taking acyclovir orally does not generally cause your blood tests to change, although one study (and only one study) showed some suggestion that red blood cells increased slightly in size during acyclovir treatment. This is not necessarily a bad thing, since the increase was not into the abnormal range. The drug does not make you sick to your stomach or cause your hair to fall out. In fact, most studies have shown no significant bad effects in people using acyclovir when compared to people using placebo (sugar pills), although the occasional person has developed allergy to it and had an allergic skin rash, which cleared up after stopping the medication.

At very high doses, administered quickly and intravenously, some patients have developed acute kidney failure. This is obviated by giving the drug slowly by vein, and this concern has never been an issue concerning oral treatment. Abnormal effects on the brain such as confusion and decreased consciousness have been occasionally seen in very complicated medical cases receiving intravenous drug. This is probably the result of drug excess caused by kidney problems and similar situations. It has also not occurred on the oral form of acyclovir.

Acyclovir has not been available long enough for scientists to consider the long-term effects past two years. Beyond that its

effects are relatively unknown; it can be considered to be neither nontoxic nor toxic. Its discovery is only a decade old, so
long-term effects in humans are, by definition, unknown. Long-
term clinical use is now extending to three or four years. No
significant problems have developed with long-term oral use,
to date. Acyclovir studies have never been done in pregnancy
or in people contemplating parenthood during the study period.
This is, therefore, another area of unknown. Mind you, during
the long-term studies so far available, no significant side effects have been seen except those minor ones noted above.
Furthermore, animals observed after taking this drug have
done pretty well on acyclovir and they have not had much in the
way of side effects. Animals who become pregnant on acyclovir
have normal offspring. At high doses (beyond those people
use), some animals have become very sick or shown decreased
sperm-making capabilities (shrunken testicle cells) and/or hair
loss. These effects were not seen in people taking the recommended doses of acyclovir. Animals do not have any increased
rates of cancer or other mutations, although some breaking of
chromosomes (the part of the cells containing the DNA) has
been noted in animals receiving very high doses.

ALTERNATIVES

As far as recurrent episodes go, aside from oral acyclovir there
has never been anything available, by prescription or otherwise, that has these types of predicted beneficial effects on
herpes simplex infections. Nevertheless, most people will not
need specific treatment when episodes are mild and short-
lived. When sores are uncomfortable, they can be soothed by
using a warm, moist cloth to soak them for a few minutes several times per day, followed by blowing dry with a hair dryer on
a low setting.

Specific and effective topical agents (creams, for example)
are under development. None that are available now are useful.
Topical acyclovir (Zovirax®) has no beneficial use for treatment or for prevention of genital herpes recurrences. There
are drugs in the offing, however, with great clinical potential as

topically applied agents. It is not the intention of this section to list all other agents being tested, although a more definitive discussion is available later in the chapter.

DOES RESISTANCE DEVELOP TO ACYCLOVIR?

This very important question has not been completely answered. In fact, resistant virus strains, which are not susceptible to acyclovir, have developed. It is the true relevance of these resistant strains that is at question.

There are basically two means by which herpes simplex virus can develop resistance to acyclovir. The first involves the enzyme thymidine kinase (TK) which is discussed above. Since acyclovir is not activated without TK, should the virus lose its TK, it also loses its susceptibility to this drug. This type of change develops readily in the laboratory setting and has also been seen to partially develop in some patients during acyclovir oral prophylaxis of genital herpes. Because acyclovir does not really have any effect on latent infection in the ganglion, however, this altered resistance does not appear to be permanent. In other words, resistance may reduce the effectiveness of acyclovir on one recurrent episode, but so far this has not been a permanent change. Next recurrence, the virus, which starts fresh from the ganglion, is susceptible to acyclovir once again. The question that has not been answered is whether this partially resistant virus would stay partially resistant if transmitted *de novo* to another individual, since that would then become the strain that establishes the new latent infection in the other individual.

The second mechanism of resistance to acyclovir results from changes in the viral DNA polymerase. Clinically, very few instances of resistance from mutations of the viral DNA polymerase have occurred (two, to be precise). These have been limited to patients with severe immune problems (bone marrow transplantation).

It will be critically important for scientists to maintain close surveillance on the resistance question as acyclovir becomes more widely used. So far, it looks like a minimal problem, but this is said only holding one's breath. Investigators continue to monitor this resistance question. For the time being, resistance is *not* a concern for the average person taking oral acyclovir.

ANY OTHER PROBLEMS?

A quick word about antibodies. These are one of the ways the body uses to fight off active herpes. Antibodies help to heal sores and may help to prevent some people from getting sores in the first place. The body triggers itself to make these antibodies in its own defense. It is not unexpected, therefore, that any drug which minimizes the amount of virus on the attack will cause a decreased amount of counter-response. Thus, Drs. Ashley and Corey found only 30 percent of patients receiving intravenous acyclovir made one specific virus antibody they measured, called vp66, while 100 percent of persons receiving placebo made this antibody within the first 30 days of their primary. If people did not make it on the first go-round, they made vp66 and the other antibodies on their first recurrence. Drs. Bernstein, Lovett, and Bryson from UCLA have published similar findings in a study of oral acyclovir, in which the quantity of "neutralizing" antiherpes antibody was reduced by treatment.

Since reduction of immunity is probably the result of decreasing the virus load on the immune system, these observations may not be a reflection of any problem. Nevertheless, they need to be considered—since when tampering with not only the virus but also the body's immunity to the virus, we are not really sure of what all of this means in the clinical setting. Once again, we are left with waiting to see what the future holds. So far, taken by themselves, antibody reductions are *probably not* a reason to avoid the drug.

SHOULD I OR SHOULDN'T I?

It goes without saying that you are the only person who can make up your own mind. Although ultimately it is a personal choice, you should decide in conjunction with your physician. In preparation for these discussions, it is a useful exercise to weigh the benefits and risks in order to help you decide if taking acyclovir is worth it for you. The government licensing bodies, which have given their stamp of approval to this agent, have not decided for you that you should or must take this drug. They have only said that it passed enough of its prelicensing tests to receive the right to be sold by prescription. The rest is up to you and your physician.

On the positive side, this is the first drug to become available that shortens recurrences as well as first episodes. Taken prophylactically it markedly and predictably reduces episode frequency. It has few, if any, significant short-term side effects at prescribed doses for up to two years (the period studied so far).

On the negative side, the mechanism of action of this drug is based upon its conversion to a DNA poison, which occurs mainly, but not exclusively, in virus-infected cells. Furthermore, because this drug is effective only when taken internally, it is not possible to deliver its effects only to the areas that need it on the skin. Nevertheless, because of its virus-dependent mechanism of action, it is *chemically* directed mainly to the affected areas. Still, all of our cells, from the nose to the toes, including heart, liver, kidney, and bone marrow, are being bathed by acyclovir with every dose ingested. So far, animal tests, human clinical trials, and widespread clinical use of this drug over the first several years have shown an excellent record of safety. Indeed, the safety record of acyclovir is greater than that of many other treatments used for other diseases. With a few exceptions at very high doses in animals, the predictive factors are good ones. Yet only availability of this drug to a large number of people, over a long period of time, will truly determine its safety in the long term. Nothing except theory points to any danger whatsoever.

The theory, however, is quite specific. When talking about changes in DNA, three major areas of concern might be raised (all of which have been and continue to be carefully tested and all of which so far continue to suggest that acyclovir is safe): teratogenesis, oncogenesis, and mutagenesis. In English, this basically translates as birth defects and cancer formation. In humans, the drug has never been tested in the setting of pregnancy. It should not be taken during pregnancy, especially early pregnancy. Presumably, most people taking this drug, however, will be having sex, and since sex has been known to cause pregnancy, words of caution are provided. Avoid getting pregnant or causing someone else to get pregnant until several weeks after stopping the drug. Why wait? No special reason. The drug is pretty much cleared from the system within a day of stopping it, although if minute quantities were sticking around in cells, these would not be detected by the tests presently available, so it might be best to wait some time.

Before answering for yourself whether you should take acyclovir you must first decide how it might benefit you. For example, if you are having a painful primary episode with swollen glands, difficulty with urination, headache, etc., a ten-day course of oral acyclovir would make you feel better up to one week earlier! Because of this and the suggestion that it might reduce recurrences in the long term, using acyclovir during a first episode, as early as possible, is definitely a good idea. By contrast, if you get one mild recurrence of genital herpes per year, it would be of minimal use to you. Figuring out where you stand on the spectrum of severity is not easy when you are the only one having your own problem. On an objective scale, you will greatly benefit from taking oral acyclovir if:

1. You are having a first episode, especially if associated with lesion pain or lymph node pain requiring pain relief, or problems urinating or headache. You would use ten days of acyclovir 200 mg five times per day. Use two capsules five times per day for your first day. Then one capsule five times per day. Continue treatment until sores are healed.
2. You are having frequently recurrent herpes episodes that you are sure are herpes each time (not chronic yeast infections, for example). Furthermore, you've had this frequency

rate sustained for quite a while (say, six months to a year or more). In addition, the episodes are very bothersome, i.e., either they hurt quite a bit or upset you or your relationship quite a bit.

Under these circumstances you could try one capsule twice a day. If this is not effective you could go up to two capsules twice per day. Other effective doses are four capsules once per day or one capsule three to five times per day, depending on what works best. For now, don't use more than five capsules a day on a chronic basis. You can expect the majority of your recurrences to be thwarted by this treatment, although you might still get tingles or other warnings which you should, for now, consider to be short recurrences. They will probably disappear after six months or so. Acyclovir suppression is effective for preventing both Type 1 and Type 2 herpes infections on all skin areas.

Once you stop this drug, you will get sores at about the same frequency as before. In some people, they come more often or feel slightly different in the period right after you stop the drug, but most times they are just as before. If possible, try to limit your periods of prophylaxis to those where you need to be free of lesions.

3. You have recurrent herpes and moderate to severe eczema requiring treatment. I would prefer to use acyclovir here because of the risk of autoinoculation of herpes to areas of involved skin. If outbreaks are frequent, I would encourage you to use acyclovir for suppression. If infrequent, I would encourage you to use acyclovir as soon as you get your warning of the next outbreak.

4. Erythema multiforme caused by herpes should also be treated with acyclovir either on a chronic or intermittent basis, depending on the frequency rate. If acyclovir does not fully prevent the skin rash, your doctor may want you to take other medication as well.

5. If you have AIDS and herpes, you should be taking oral acyclovir as a suppressive regimen to avoid serious complications. The same is true for other types of immuno-

compromise, such as leukemia and transplantation. Your doctor can guide you about when you should take acyclovir.

What if your recurrent herpes is neither frequent nor severe? Then your choice about whether to use oral acyclovir falls into a gray zone. In other words, you should reach your own decision after considering the facts:

1. Treating recurrences of herpes. Taking acyclovir shortens your episodes by about a day. They still cycle forward to healing as before only they're slightly shorter. They itch and tingle just the same for just as long as before. They still have virus in them during active phases of infection. The gain is slight. The cost will be about $0.60 to $0.70 per capsule (U.S. funds). The drug is still taken internally. Are your recurrences infrequent, but very long and painful? Then taking acyclovir may be more helpful. Do you get a bad headache or leg ache that bothers you a lot? Then it might be worth a try, although it is not clear that these symptoms will be benefited by taking acyclovir. In contrast, are you like most people with herpes in that your recurrences generally last five to six days and feel about as painful as a mosquito bite? Then why treat them with a systemic (taken internally) drug? Your gain is going to be very slight. Why not wait a couple of more years for an effective topical agent and meanwhile treat your sores symptomatically, if necessary, as described earlier?

2. Treating mild first episodes of herpes. The less severe the problem, the less the gain from treatment. The medical literature is not so clear on this point as an indication for acyclovir. Early in a first clinical episode, neither the physician nor the patient can accurately determine whether an episode is a true primary or not. A single, mild sore could develop into a serious primary after a few days. Thus, unless the physician can instantly perform the antibody test required to differentiate primary from nonprimary initial episodes, he or she should probably treat any first episode with oral acyclovir as soon as treatment can be begun.

3. Preventing less frequent herpes recurrences by daily prophylaxis. What is the cutoff point? Obviously, daily systemic treatment to prevent one episode a year is not worth it. Often, preventing three episodes per month is worth it. A generally held cutoff would be in the neighborhood of one recurrence every four to six weeks, or more frequently. It must depend on you, of course, but if you gain 5 days of being lesion-free for every 50, this represents only 10 percent of the time. For every 100 days we're talking 5 percent of the time, and so on. Nevertheless, it's tempting to take a pill and feel one is regaining control of one's body! This is not a cure, however, so try to think it out—what will your control gain for you? Even taking acyclovir every day will not usually prevent all outbreaks, nor will it totally eliminate the possibility of shedding of virus from skin.

4. "Special events" are another use for this agent. Let's say you only get one outbreak every couple of months, but you are just beginning a new relationship, or experiencing an unusual amount of stress at work, or due for your first vacation in two years, or whatever scenario fits. Oral acyclovir offers control over herpes when you need it. If you use acyclovir for special events, take it as for suppression—i.e., before an outbreak has begun, for a predetermined length of time. When the event is over, you may stop using acyclovir.

5. You may consider acyclovir if your occupation requires it. For example, if you get fairly frequent whitlows (finger infections) and you are a bartender or a dentist or a grocery clerk, acyclovir may keep you employed. This is an important use for some people.

6. Preventing herpes in someone who has never had it will not be discussed in the drug monograph since the study testing it for this has never been tried. Yet it will be tempting. Should you allow yourself to be tempted? It is a guess that acyclovir orally might, in some people, prevent herpes infections after transmission has occurred, but before latent infection has been established. It has done so in some animals tested. In some clinical cases, it has definitely failed to do so and in some it has probably succeeded. This will

likely never be studied in humans because of ethical questions. Nevertheless, if you realize *after* you start making love that you have a wet lesion in an active phase, you could discuss with your partner and your partner's physician the possibility of having your partner use acyclovir orally for five or ten days in the *hopes* of preventing infection. If your partner has never had herpes and exposure was fairly certain, he or she might wish to try it. This is unproven and untested. While I cannot recommend this approach on the basis of scientific evidence, the risk-to-benefit ratio could be very much in favor of taking acyclovir for this, depending on the situation. Talk to your own physician.

What about your unaffected partner taking this drug all the time? This is *not* recommended, although one can imagine it will be tried. Since it may not even work for this, exposing oneself chronically to this drug without having any evidence of infection would be fairly unwise. In this situation, the risk to benefit ratio would probably not be in your favor.

PERSONAL CONCLUSIONS

It is a great relief to have in one's medicine cabinet a partial answer to a nagging, persisting, uncomfortable problem. Control of herpes is now possible for the first time. Cure is not. But the ability to stop herpes from coming up into sores by taking a treatment, which in careful studies not only looks effective but also safe is indeed exciting news. Nevertheless, before taking acyclovir every day for the next ten years, ask yourself whether it will have been worth it if it turns out 20 years from now to have caused some long-term problem. If your answer is a definite "yes," go for it! If your answer is a definite "no," then don't. If your answer is "I don't know," then you have a harder decision to make. So far, with three or four years of clinical experience, this drug continues to look *very* safe. If you feel that you need it, and you can afford to take it, then you can *probably* make that decision with minimal concern. We're making fast strides ahead, you know. The next couple of years could produce effective topical treatment or even some other approach.

If you're not in a hurry, you will have nothing to lose by waiting. I hope this helps you to decide.

What does the future hold?

The field of drug therapy against herpes has rapidly progressed over the last few years. During 1982, we saw the first proven effective therapy for primary genital herpes—topical acyclovir—achieve government approval and appear in the drug stores. By 1985, oral acyclovir became available on prescription. The number of herpes researchers all over the world has increased dramatically, possibly with more rapidity than the incidence of the infection itself. Pharmaceutical firms have joined in the herpes battle, each one hoping for a chance to have the best therapy for herpes.

Many objective targets for therapy are used to assess the usefulness of a drug. The herpes researcher uses buzz words such as "double-blind," "randomized," "controlled," "time to total healing," "virus titer," "time of virus shedding," "pain scores," "itching scores," "patient-initiated therapy," and "clinic-initiated therapy." This list is nearly endless. These words are descriptions for different end points used to measure drug effects or for different methods of conducting a human drug test, often called a "clinical trial." Today, in studying genital herpes, a new drug will be considered to be effective only if it can satisfy some basic tests:

1. It must be safe and effective at killing virus *in vitro*—in the test tube.
2. It must be safe and effective in helping animals experimentally infected with herpes. Some drugs are not intended to kill the herpes virus, per se, but rather to boost the body's natural immunity. These drugs would be ineffective in the test tube, but would have to show an effect in the animal model.
3. It must be studied for use in herpes in a double-blind, placebo-controlled, randomized trial. The trial is called double-blind because both the patient and the investigator

are blind as to which patient is getting which therapy, i.e., neither knows which volunteer is getting the real drug and which volunteer is getting a placebo (pill without the drug) until the end of the trial. The placebo control drug is one which looks like, tastes like, and smells like the real drug (except it does not contain the real drug). The study is randomized by a statistician, so that there is no possible way to predict which volunteer might receive the real drug.

In the clinical trial a person with herpes uses the new test drug. Factors that might reveal if the drug is useful are monitored very closely, for example, the appearance of sores, the duration of sores, the pain and itching of sores, or the duration of virus in sores.

Certain things that are "known" to affect the course of the illness are grouped together for study. For example, since recurrent herpes lasts about one week and primary herpes about three, it is clear that the experiences of primary and recurrent herpes should not be compared to each other. Rather, they must be separately studied. Other factors also affect the outcome of a study.

Results of the drug testing are tabulated and then locked into a computer. Once the results are locked in an unchangeable fashion, the code is broken. Then the statisticians and scientists and physicians can analyze whether the people who got the drug responded in a way that is different from the group who got the look-alike, smell-alike, taste-alike placebo. Then, and only then, if the drug works better than the placebo, one can draw conclusions about whether the drug will be useful or not. If the good effect is clear, in mathematical terms, this is called "statistically significant." This means the effect of the drug is unlikely to have occurred as a result of chance alone.

Many drugs, chemicals, natural substances, food additives, solvents, methods of biofeedback, hypnosis, acupuncture, and so forth have been purported to work for herpes. Of the ones tested in a carefully designed double-blind, placebo-controlled, randomized clinical trial, however, only a handful show any positive effects. These drugs and some others will be discussed further. Indeed, as far as antiherpes drug therapy goes, the present and the future are beginning to overlap. We are actively discovering new chemicals to kill the virus and also new ways in which to use those chemicals.

Any infection results from an imbalance between the number of infecting particles (the invasion size) and the immune defense network. Drugs for herpes are being developed to affect both sides of the network. We might try to boost the body's natural defenses—in other words, boost immunity. Then the body might kill the virus faster or keep it latent more effectively. Alternatively, we can develop drugs to actively kill the virus, as penicillin kills gonorrhea.

DRUGS TO KILL THE VIRUS (ANTIVIRAL AGENTS)

Thymidine analogs

As already outlined, acyclovir works on the basis of its chemical similarity to thymidine. A number of other agents work by a similar fashion.

Several derivatives of acyclovir that might improve on acyclovir's absorption characteristics or potency are being examined in animals. One such derivative is 6-deoxyacyclovir. This chemical is much better absorbed by mouth than is acyclovir, making it possible to achieve much higher drug levels after taking capsules. This agent is converted by a human enzyme called xanthine oxidase to acyclovir. Since xanthine oxidase is everywhere in the body, this conversion takes place readily. Once converted to acyclovir, this drug should theoretically work the same as taking acyclovir, except more will be available to do the job.

Another acyclovir derivative is ganciclovir (DHPG, 1, 3-dihydroxy-2-propoxymethyl guanine 2'-NDG, BW759). The people responsible for synthesizing this drug report that it is 68 times as effective against herpes as acyclovir given orally to mice. That means nothing now to those of us without tails, but a few years from now that may turn out to be a very important number. Unfortunately, this agent can inhibit the formation of sperm at levels much lower than required for acyclovir to do the same. This makes the drug somewhat impractical for herpes simplex right now. However, another herpes virus, cytomegalovirus, is very susceptible to this agent. Ganciclovir will likely find its niche there.

Ethyldeoxyuridine (EDU, edoxudine, Aedurid®, Virostat®) is also undergoing active testing. This drug is now sold in Germany and preliminary reports show it to be effective there. These studies were small and not controlled, however. This drug is being actively studied in North America now in large, double-blind, controlled trials as a topical agent (cream). Early data show that this agent is very effective at reducing the period of virus shedding. It also reduces the signs (tenderness of lesions, swelling of lesions) in women. This is a step forward in the topical treatment of recurrent infection. The drug might become generally available in Canada in the next couple of years.

At the Seventh International Congress of Virology held in August 1987, Dr. M. R. Boyd of Beecham Pharmaceuticals reported on the effects of a compound designated BRL39123. This is a close relative of acyclovir, but holds certain potential advantages in terms of its mechanism of action and its ease of administration. This agent will be receiving a lot of attention in the genital herpes arena over the next few years. Keep your eye on this one.

Phosphonoformic acid (foscarnet, Foscavir®)

Foscarnet is a small chemical that works by very different mechanisms from the thymidine analogs. It does not depend on TK at all. Rather, because of its small size, it gets into all kinds of cells, infected or not. It also penetrates skin without much difficulty. Foscarnet is also an enzyme-inhibitor. The enzyme it has chosen to interrupt is called DNA polymerase. We discussed DNA before—the hereditary material made up of code sequences of four chemicals. It is DNA polymerase that tells these four chemicals to start building the DNA chain. It is like a "start and keep going" button. Herpes has its own DNA polymerase and cells have their own. Foscarnet is a much more potent inhibitor of viral DNA polymerase than of cellular DNA polymerase. This drug has recently been tested in Sweden, where it was shown to decrease the time that lesions were not healed in recurrent herpes from 5.0 days to 4.0 days. This positive effect was seen more in men than in women. In this study, women also healed faster, but the differences were not statistically significant. Side effects were observed in men at a cream concentration of one percent. These adverse effects included irritation and occasional ulceration at the site of drug application.

Adverse effects have been avoided by reducing the concentration of this agent in the cream. A recent Canadian study in seven centers showed a good antiviral effect from the cream in men. Symptoms were slightly reduced after the first day of treatment. However, the times to healing and the duration of symptoms, overall, were not improved. This negative outcome for foscarnet demonstrates the need for large and well-defined studies before drawing conclusions about any new agent.

Miscellaneous Compounds

Another interesting group of chemicals which were developed at the Sloan-Kettering Cancer Institute are showing some promise. FIAC (fluoro-iodoaracytosine) is the name for the extremely potent parent drug. The ethyl form, FEAU, has been quite effective in animal models of genital herpes. Studies have also shown benefits from this compound in treating certain types of hepatitis in animals. Human studies have not been performed.

IMMUNITY BOOSTERS

Interferon

You might have heard of interferon as the miracle cure for cancer that still has a long way to go. Interferon originally got its name back in 1957 because it "interfered" with viruses. Now it has become reasonably inexpensive to make this drug in bacteria using recombinant DNA tricks. Active testing against herpes is underway in clinical trials. This might take the form of active treatment for new sores or daily or weekly prevention shots. We already know that one type of interferon can suppress oral herpes outbreaks if taken just before the outbreak. The trick is to know when the outbreak is coming.

Results of clinical trials using systemic interferon for genital herpes have shown conflicting results. In general, the side effects are too severe to warrant its general use. On the other hand, use of interferon in a gel preparation is not associated with significant side effects. In a recent multicenter study, reported at the 1987 International Congress of Virology, topical high-dose recombinant interferon displayed a good antiviral effect, along with some clinical benefit in the treatment of recurrent herpes. Studies of topically applied interferon, in a cream, where it has been combined with the spermicidal agent nonoxynol-9 are also showing some promise. These two agents in combination work together in their antiviral action. This laboratory phenomenon (called synergy) *might* translate into good clinical benefit. Early published results are quite positive. Properly controlled and monitored, double-blind, placebo-controlled trials are ongoing. The results are not yet known.

Inosiplex

Inosiplex (Isoprinosine®) has a direct antiherpes effect in the test tube. Furthermore, it has been shown to increase lymphocyte transformation against herpes simplex virus. In other words, one can measure a laboratory effect that shows that lymphocytes (see Chapter 2) in people receiving this drug get more excited and more active around herpes than they do in people not receiving inosiplex.

In 1972 Drs. Steinberg and Ruiz reported the results of a double-blind, controlled study in a Mexican medical journal. This showed that patients receiving inosiplex healed their herpes in 5.2 days as opposed to 9.0 days for placebo recipients. Both oral and genital herpes were studied, but not separately. Primary and recurrent herpes were not kept separate in their analysis. Furthermore, virus cultures were not routinely performed to document herpes infection.

The next year a report by Drs. Chang, Fuimara, and Weinstein at the Interscience Conference on Antimicrobial Agents and Chemotherapy suggested that this drug could be useful in primary herpes. Their double-blind, placebo-controlled trial did not suggest any effect on recurrent herpes, nor any effect on the rate of recurrences. In 1975, Drs. Wickett and Bradshaw presented results of a study of 53 patients. They concluded from their double-blind, placebo-controlled trial that this drug shortens the course of a herpes outbreak. Once again, the most critical error of study design possible was present in this study, in that persons with both primary and recurrent herpes were analyzed together. As we already know, primary herpes may last for up to three weeks as opposed to seven to ten days for recurrent herpes. In fact, in assessing their result one notes that twice as many primary patients are included in their placebo group. In other words, the people one expects to be having longer outbreaks are having their outbreaks averaged in with the placebo results. Then one compares placebo and drug, and the drug looks great. Is this because the drug is effective or because one has compared apples to oranges?

Another study from Paris, France, has suggested in a double-blind, placebo-controlled trial that inosiplex may be effective in recurrent herpes. In this study, where virus cultures were not obtained, lesions dried up by day three in over 50 percent of the drug recipients and only 25 percent of placebo recipients. In a letter to the editor of *The Lancet*, Dr. M. Galli and his coworkers from Milan, Italy, have reported the results of giving inosiplex to 31 people with genital herpes. These people were treated for one week at a time on four separate occasions. Herpes recurrences declined from the year before treatment to the year after, but this effect could not be attributed to the influence of the drug.

This agent has so far been associated with one side effect, the elevation of uric acid levels in the blood. Uric acid is a metabolite of the drug (a breakdown product) and this elevation is not surprising, nor especially worrisome.

Inosiplex is an interesting drug worthy of further study. All too often, it has been the unfortunate victim of less than optimal study design. Some of these trials have left more questions than answers. Until the results of properly controlled trials are in, inosiplex should not be used for herpes.

Other immunity boosters

There is one more important class of future drugs to be discussed called pyrimidinones. These drugs do nothing harmful to herpes in the test tube. When painted on the skin of a guinea pig they somehow resist herpes infection. There is more to find out here, since nobody really knows why it works. On the other hand, the effects in animals have been interesting. Clinical trials with these agents may soon be in the offing.

Cimetidine (Tagamet®) has been used in six patients by Dr. Wakefield from New South Wales, Australia. He reports a reduction in episode frequency but fails to use a placebo in his study. He has compared the changes before and after treatment solely on the basis of the patient's recall of episode frequency. Again, no conclusions can be drawn.

Vaccines

Herpes vaccines have actually been around for a while. In some European countries, vaccines (Lupidon-G®) are generally available. There has always been some concern about their safety because herpes in a killed form, such as is present in the vaccine, still has its DNA. This might be a concern in terms of inducing cancer. Despite these reservations, many people are attracted to these "whole virus vaccines" because they have a reported capability to induce a 70 to 80 percent "improvement rate" in frequency and severity of recurrences. These studies were not controlled and are not generally accepted. There are no good data on risks with this vaccine. Because there is no *proven* positive effect and no proven safety record, the vaccine is not approved in the United States or Canada.

Recently, however, some progress has been made in finding which part of the virus was important in giving immunity. These parts that induce immunity, also known as "subunits," can be purified and given as a vaccine, thus theoretically circumventing the problem with possible safety risks. Subunit vaccines are now being produced for clinical trials. It may also become possible to effectively change the living virus enough to create a live vaccine. This might be more effective at inducing good immunity because it is living. Using special DNA techniques the virus genes could be changed so that herpes loses its ability to cause cancer or its ability to form latent infection, etc. Then this altered strain could be safely administered to people. This work is still theoretical.

Certain vaccines can effectively protect mice or guinea pigs *before* infection. They also effectively result in antibody production in humans. But why should any vaccine be useful to *treat* recurrent herpes? People with herpes already have antibody and other types of immunity to herpes. As far as we can tell, people with herpes have normal amounts of antibody and normal lymphocyte responses to herpes. So what will vaccine-induced increases in immunity accomplish? Will this alter the course of recurrences? There is no good clinical reason to think that vaccines will do anything for the person who already has established infection. On the other hand, vaccines may turn out to be very useful for the general population. In other words, if we could give everyone an effective vaccine in early childhood, then there may be enough immune protection to make it more difficult for an unaffected person to get herpes. If this occurs, the risks would decrease. This is more likely to be helpful for our children and their children than for us.

Regardless, trying vaccines (once they are made safe or more effective) will be worth a try in recurrent herpes. They might also play a role in prevention for partners or others at high risk for getting herpes. Early results of the first American clinical trials were recently reported. This vaccine was not effective. Final results will require very careful interpretation. New vaccines are under development and advances in vaccine engineering are occurring rapidly. The future of vaccines for herpes remains an unanswered question for now.

What are the alternative treatments?

Alternatives to standard medical therapy have been present ever since there were accepted standards. These alternatives are most popular when standard therapies are inadequate. Until recently, with the advent of new and effective specific antiherpes drug therapy, alternatives were all that was available for someone who wanted to do something specifically therapeutic for herpes.

Some of the alternative chemicals listed here are not drugs in the legal sense. A drug in the legal sense has to undergo rigorous testing before it is allowed to be licensed and sold for physicians to prescribe. In order to gain the license, the drug must be shown to be effective in the treatment of the disease for which it is being recommended. Next, it must be safe enough that the treatment effect is considered better than its side effects. Alternative drugs and chemicals do not necessarily fit these criteria, however, making some of them possible to obtain without fulfilling these criteria. Some reasons that alternative chemicals may remain available are as follows:

1. The chemical was given drug status before the laws giving government control came into effect, i.e., these drugs comply with the "grandfather clause."
2. The chemical is considered safe without testing because it is a food by-product. An example is L-lysine.
3. The chemical is considered safe because it is an "accepted" food additive. BHT is an example here.
4. The chemical is licensed by another government, for example in a European country, and imported for personal use.

It is important to realize that just because you are able to buy a chemical that someone says you can take as medicine does not necessarily mean that anyone knows it is safe or effective. It is only tested for safety and efficacy if it is called a drug and taken through drug clearance channels[1]. BHT and L-lysine, among others, have never been shown to be safe or effective in humans in the doses being recommended by some people for herpes. Nevertheless, just like drugs in the pharmacy, these chemicals go into the body, circulate in the blood, deposit in body tissue, and so on. The only difference is that we do not always know if these chemicals are safe at the doses used, and their usefulness in terms of positive effects is unknown.

When it comes to specific antiherpes treatments, the list of potential alternative approaches is very long. We often seek easy answers, which address mainly our hopes of cure, rather than answers that require painfully long adherence to difficult rules. Alternative treatments are fraught with potential dangers. For example, if alternatives are sought in lieu of standard treatments for a life-threatening, but potentially curable disease, needless deaths may result. Happily, this is not the case with herpes, because it is not normally life-threatening. Yet simplistic answers to difficult problems can harm the person victimized. It can rob the person of money, time, and even hope. Be selective and careful when choosing alternative therapies or standard therapies. The alternatives arousing the greatest interest are listed below. This is not intended to be a complete list.

Butylated Hydroxytoluene (BHT)

BHT is a food additive. The chemical is synthesized from two organic compounds, called p-cresol and isobutylene. It cannot be dissolved in water, but is easily dissolved in organic solvents such as alcohol and gasoline. BHT is literally every-

[1]Even then, some of the older drugs and drug combinations commonly used and prescribed are not considered effective. There is an excellent book on this subject which you are encouraged to read, if interested: *Pills That Don't Work* by S. M. Wolfe, M.D., and C. M. Coley (New York: Farrar Straus & Giroux, 1981).

where. In 1976, Americans consumed, by mouth, nearly nine million pounds of the stuff. BHT hides in margarine, instant potatoes, and chewing gum, to mention only a few. It is fed to chickens and other animals and lives with us daily. We consume 1 to 2 mg each per day. Each American has on the average 1.3 ± 0.82 parts per million in body fat.

BHT kills herpes simplex virus in the laboratory. When dissolved in mineral oil at a concentration of 5 percent or 15 percent and applied to the skin of hairless mice infected with herpes simplex virus Type 1, BHT was better than mineral oil alone at reducing the number of herpes lesions. BHT is probably a virus envelope interrupter. In other words, it can kill viruses that depend on having an envelope because it may dissolve the envelope. Certainly other mechanisms are also possible. Two important criteria in drug testing have been satisfied in the testing of BHT as an antiherpes treatment:

1. It kills herpes simplex virus in the test tube.
2. It is effective at speeding the healing of sores in some animal models (mouse) when applied to the skin in mineral oil. Not all investigators agree.

As a topically applied mixture in mineral oil, BHT therapy also resulted in skin reddening and some skin sloughing. This agent has never been reported to have been given by mouth to animals for treatment of herpes. Despite this, it is being discussed in a recent popular book[2] at doses ranging from 250 mg per day to as much as 2,000 mg per day in the treatment of herpes. There are no published data anywhere in the scientific literature on the safety of this type of agent being administered in these doses to humans. Because we take BHT every day as a food additive, this compound is "presumed safe." However, these doses are as much as 1,000 times the usual daily intake. At even higher doses the following things happen to animals in experiments (not a complete list):

[2]Durk Pearson and Sandy Shaw, *Life Extension: A Practical Scientif* *Approach* (New York: Warner Books, 1982).

- LAF$_1$ mice given an otherwise improper and incomplete synthetic diet lived longer if the diet was supplemented with BHT.
- BHT did not affect the life span of C57BL/6J mice who were given proper nutrition, although it did seem to partially reverse the hazardous effects of inadequate nutrition.
- BHT prolonged the life span of BALB/c mice who began supplementing their diet with BHT at 11 weeks of age. It was of less benefit if started earlier in life.
- At higher doses, it can cause animals to bleed into the brain or even bleed to death.
- It can damage heart cells.
- It can retard weight gain.
- It can decrease the metabolism of the adrenal glands.
- It can cause disorganization and destructive changes of lung cells and can lead to serious lung damage.
- The liver becomes enlarged, a phenomenon that disappears when the agent is stopped. A system of liver enzymes called the P-450 system is induced. (If this system stays induced for prolonged periods it will change the way other drugs and natural products are metabolized. For example, if vitamin D is metabolized more quickly by induced enzymes, over a period of time a vitamin deficiency might develop that can lead to a bone disease called osteomalacia.)

Most of the effects of BHT, both "good" and "bad," occur at high doses, much higher than the amounts we ingest incidentally every day. However, the long-term effects of even the small doses that we use are poorly understood. Indeed, the wisdom of ingesting even these small amounts might well be questioned. There have been no human studies at these doses with BHT for herpes treatment or for safety. On the other hand, this chemical has passed the preliminaries in terms of developing a new antiherpes drug—it works in the test tube and, at least in some investigators' hands, on the skin of animals. It was next tried *on the skin* of humans in a trial conducted by Dr. S. Spruance from the University of Utah. This double-blind, placebo-controlled trial failed to show any significant benefit from using topical BHT. At this point there is no precedent for humans to ingest BHT orally in these doses. Orally, it should be best avoided until more information becomes available. Topically, it is not helpful.

L-lysine

L-lysine is a naturally occurring substance called an amino acid. Amino acids are the building blocks for all proteins. Proteins in the body are used to make the structure that holds us up and the molecular array that runs our metabolic processes. Our bodies have immense control over amino acids because we depend on them so much. We are constantly making and destroying amino acids and interconnecting them one to the other in order to maintain the exquisite balance—just so.

Nearly 20 years ago, an effect of L-lysine against herpes simplex virus was noted in the test tube. It seems that changing the nutritional environment of herpes alters its capability to make its essential proteins. This amino acid balance can be critical, especially between two amino acids, lysine and arginine. These work in a somewhat opposing manner, in that lysine in *excessive* amounts damages the virus, while arginine, if *deprived* from the culture media, has a similar effect. People talk about the lysine/arginine ratio as the important factor. There is little doubt that a high ratio will have a negative influence on herpes simplex virus in culture. It is a giant leap to say that altering these chemicals in the diet will change your ability to combat clinical infection. In fact, it is not known whether this ratio can be changed in the body. There have been clinical trials with L-lysine, though they have never involved total dietary management as is being suggested by a number of the L-lysine advocates. The lysine work to date in humans is summarized below.

Dr. R.S. Griffith and his coworkers published an article in 1978 describing a multicenter trial of L-lysine for herpes infections. Doses of 300 mg to 1,000 mg per day were used. A long-term beneficial effect was observed. However, this study had no control group. Yet, many people with herpes swear by L-lysine. Recently, popular trade magazines have attested to this fact. It has also been clearly and scientifically established that without proper controls, however, placebo effects are quite profound. In one study, 77 percent of 26 patients reported their oral herpes lesions to be markedly reduced in severity and duration by treatment with water! Ether, which was the test substance in that clinical trial was shown to be no more effective than the water placebo. Back to L-lysine. If water works for 77 percent of people who think they are using a drug, then it would be wise to be very critical of studies that have no control group.

Two controlled trials of L-lysine have been performed in Denmark by Dr. N. Milman and his coworkers. First, L-lysine was used as treatment for oral herpes recurrent attacks. Treatment took place immediately upon sensing a coming recurrence. This was tested on 251 recurrences. There was clearly no beneficial effect when used in this fashion. Next, patients with recurrent oral herpes were given 1,000 mg daily for 12 weeks. The control group received starch powder tablets. After 12 weeks, the groups switched places. One can argue strongly about the statistical validity of such a switch. Regardless, the patients in each group had herpes recurrences. There was no effect of the drug on the number of recurrences, the rate of recurrences, the rate of healing of recurrences, or the symptoms of recurrences. Fourteen patients had no recurrences at all during lysine treatment, whereas four patients had no recurrences during starch treatment. This was considered to be of "borderline significance."

Another more recent study came from the Dermatology Branch at the National Institutes of Health in Bethesda, Maryland. Drs. J. DiGiovanna and H. Blank performed a randomized, double-blind, placebo-controlled trial of L-lysine taken for four to five months. The drug was given as 400 mg three times daily. All persons were advised not to take "excessive" amounts of seeds, nuts, or chocolate because of their arginine content. Their article entitled "Failure of lysine in frequently recurrent herpes simplex infection" was published in the January 1984 edition of *Archives of Dermatology*. No substantial benefits of treatment were noted, although only

20 patients were studied and follow-up during the treatment period was left mostly up to the patients themselves. This leaves interpretations somewhat difficult. Nevertheless, all participants had a positive diagnosis made at the time of entry and no beneficial effects were seen.

In conclusion, we do not know whether the lysine/arginine ratio matters for herpes in the human. We have only recently seen any dietary controls as part of the experimental design, and in this setting no benefits were noted. We do not know if altering the amino acid intake actually changes the nutrients available to the virus inside the cell. Knowing the safeguards in the system against tampering with such important building blocks, it seems doubtful to me that much actually changes inside of the cell. We are also in the dark concerning the safety of this regimen. Because amino acids are "natural" nutrients, they can be put into tablets and sold for consumption at any dosage. However, alterations of amino acids have undetermined effects on the body. Unfortunately, because these are not called drugs, they are not controlled as drugs. We may never know.

2-Deoxy-D-Glucose (2-DG)

Glucose is simple sugar. Cells and viruses use simple sugar for a number of different processes. 2-DG is an analog of glucose. It is a look-alike as far as the metabolic system is concerned, so a cell needing a glucose molecule might grab and try to use a 2-DG molecule instead if one were around to grab. When viruses grab 2-DG they seem to put the molecule into the virus envelope. This effectively antagonizes herpes simplex growth by creating a useless envelope. A lot of excitement was stirred up by a report in a June 1979 issue of the *Journal of the American Medical Association* stating that human genital herpes infections could be effectively treated with this agent applied in a topical cream. The investigators claimed that using this cream decreased the severity of the disease while it was being used, and, furthermore, that it decreased the rate of subsequent recurrences.

This study has come under intense criticism. In the study

the numbers of placebo patients was very small. In recurrent herpes episodes, the *average* number of days to healing of lesions was 12.0 after the placebo patients started using the cream, which occurred on average four days after the onset of symptoms. In other words, the healing time of the placebo group for a recurrence of herpes was more than two weeks. This is indeed an extraordinary period. When compared to the treatment group who had healing times of 6.8 days (plus the four days before using the cream) there was a great statistical difference. This means that drug recipients healed in 6.8 to 10.8 days, a standard and expected duration for an untreated recurrence. The reasons for the very long placebo group healing time are unknown. Subsequent studies in humans with this drug are not published. However, animals were tested for effect. 2-DG has been extensively tested against genital herpes in a guinea pig and in a mouse animal model. No positive effects were seen. The drug did not inhibit the development of sores, nor did it inhibit the quantity of virus present. 2-DG has been reported to be useful in rabbit eye infections with herpes simplex, although these effects are not impressive when compared to other antiviral agents.

For now, 2-DG is on the back burner. Several years have passed since the initial publication. This compound is not available for purchase or other use in the treatment of genital herpes.

Contraceptive Foam

Nonoxynol-9 is a "surfactant." It acts very similarly to soap. In the test tube, this agent, like soap, effectively inactivates herpes simplex virus. It was reported in early observations (uncontrolled) to be effective in the therapy of genital herpes infection. When tested in a placebo-controlled trial, nonoxynol-9 was not beneficial. In fact, herpes lesions in recipients of this drug healed more slowly than those in the placebo group. One company is selling surfactants as topical treatment for recurrent herpes. However, their evidence of effectiveness is not as strong as it should be. More promising data have come from using nonoxynol-9 in combination with topical interferon for treatment. This work is still in progress and is discussed in the section on interferon. Nonoxynol-9 is also a very important preventative tool, when used properly, in combination with a condom. As a prevention tool, nonoxynol-9 is safe and shows demonstrable antiviral effects in the test tube. See Chapter 12 for further information.

Lithium

Lithium satisfies the requirement of being effective against herpes in the test tube. It inactivates herpes simplex at a concentration of 30 to 60 milliequivalents. This is 20 to 60 times the levels considered appropriate for treating humans for manic depressive illness (the only clinical setting where lithium should be used).

Very few people with herpes have been reportedly helped (for herpes) by lithium. Furthermore, there are very important and potentially dangerous side effects to lithium. Regardless of how alternative you wish to be, lithium is dangerous unless under the rigid control of experts administering this agent. It should not be used for herpes unless as part of a carefully controlled clinical trial.

Zinc

Zinc is also capable of inhibiting herpes simplex virus in the test tube. It is a common component of various skin creams. Zinc has been tried as a cream combined with ultrasound treatment and has also been given by mouth. Neither of these settings, although reported in the literature, was set up as a trial with placebo controls, randomization, etc. Therefore, conclusions cannot be drawn.

Dimethyl Sulfoxide (DMSO)

This organic solvent rapidly penetrates skin. It is so effective at penetrating skin that some recipients have been able to taste it in the mouth within seconds of applying it to the skin surface. DMSO is also very effective at carrying antiviral agents with it. Thus, it has been thought that mixing a good drug in DMSO may make it penetrate better and therefore work better. Indeed, in the case of acyclovir and BVDU, DMSO does markedly enhance drug penetration through the skin of guinea pigs. DMSO has been tried clinically in the case of idoxuridine. Early reports suggested that a combination of idoxuridine with DMSO might be an effective herpes treatment. Drs. Silvestri, Corey, and Holmes, however, published an exhaustive study in the *Journal of the American Medical Association* (*JAMA*) in August 1982. Idoxuridine in DMSO was found to have no clinical effect on primary or recurrent herpes. People receiving the treatment complained of burning and allergy. One patient developed local cancer at the site of drug application. Regardless of whether this resulted from the use of the drug, DMSO is not indicated for the treatment of herpes.

Adenosine Monophosphate (AMP)

In 1979, Drs. S.H. Sklar and E. Buimovici-Klein reported that adenosine-5′-monophosphate was "effective" in the treatment of patients with recurrent oral herpes. AMP was given by intramuscular injection in 9 to 12 injections on alternate days. The authors claimed from this uncontrolled study that pain and discomfort were ameliorated quickly. AMP is a natural cellular compound. Side effects (which had not been extensively looked for) were not seen. It has been suggested that this agent might stabilize membranes in the nervous system preventing reactivation. Indeed, in a mouse model of recurring herpes simplex infection, it was suggested that this agent might be able to prevent recurrences under certain experimental conditions. Although the animal results were interesting, studies were also not placebo-controlled, making the results difficult to interpret.

A more recent consideration of this topic appeared in the March 8, 1985 issue of *JAMA*. In this article Drs. Sklar, Blue, Alexander, and Bodian demonstrated a useful effect on the treatment of herpes zoster infections (shingles). Their trial was double-blind, randomized, and placebo-controlled. Their numbers were small (32 volunteers total). The drug was put into gel and injected intramuscularly three times per week. This tells us some new and interesting information about the treatment of herpes zoster. Further clinical trials will be necessary. For now, there is nothing new on the subject of AMP and genital or oral herpes.

Other Treatments

The following agents have not yet been discussed. Space does not permit a full analysis of each. None have been reported in the scientific world as proven effective against herpes in a clinical trial using placebos and controls. Thus, their usefulness is unknown. Some have received "anecdotal" treatment in the scientific literature. In other words, they may have been suggested as possibly effective, but the numbers or the design of the experiment were not possible to evaluate. Some may be more carefully studied in the future. Others may not.

Such agents include acidophilus, acupuncture, aloe vera, antibiotics[3], application of heat, application of ice, aspirin, ginseng, herbal mixtures, hypnosis, laser therapy[3], povidone-iodine (Betadine®), red algae extract, transcendental meditation, and vitamin B complexes B12, C, and E.

[3]Potential or established side effects mean that these agents should not be used for herpes unless human experiment is part of a carefully designed, properly supervised clinical trial, which includes informed consent.

12

CONDOMS AND
SAFER SEX

...until Love Story is remade with moving episodes of condom-related sex play, the rubber sheath will continue to be associated with casual sex and fear of disease. Failure to glamourise the condom may have serious consequences.

GERMAINE GREER,
*Sex and Destiny: The Politics
of Human Fertility*

What is a condom, exactly?

The condom is a penis sheath, usually made out of latex rubber or a natural membrane from sheep intestine. Historians suggest that Gabriele Fallopio was the first to use a linen sheath as protection from syphilis. England's King Charles II was apparently the first user of the membrane prophylactic. These penis covers were made from the gastrointestinal tract of sheep or other animals. While its precise origins are not certain, many believe that Charles II's physician, Dr. Condom, designed the device to prevent undesired children from the mistresses of his king. Casanova went on to describe condom use in great detail during the eighteenth century. High cost limited their use at that time to the upper classes of Europe. By the middle of the nineteenth century, however, the process of vulcanization of rubber allowed the price of condoms to drop considerably. During the 1930s more than 300 million latex condoms were sold annually in the United States. Along came the birth control pill, the intrauterine device, and the diaphragm, and the condom business suffered. Along came genital herpes, and the condom business continued to suffer. Along came AIDS, and the condom business began to flourish.

Who should be using condoms?

So much for history. The time has come to consider strongly the use of the condom as a birth control device, which, when properly used, also prevents transmission of most sexually transmitted diseases. Let us first consider the theoretical ideal. If *every individual* used condoms, along with the **spermicidal agent nonoxynol-9** *each* time he or she had sexual intercourse until such time as both partners agreed to enter a permanent, monogamous relationship, AIDS and most other sexually transmitted diseases would begin to vanish from the earth. That is how effective these things are, *if used correctly*. Concerning genital herpes, you will note later in this chapter that I am advising that condoms be used only during the inactive phases of infection. From a *statistical* point of view, of course, they would reduce transmission even when used in the active phases. From the *individual's* point of view, however, both protected and unprotected sexual contact are not advised during active phases of herpes. Condoms are recommended for nearly everyone, then, regardless of whether genital herpes has complicated your relationship. If one partner does have genital herpes, however, the condom, properly used, may add a new and very attractive element to the relationship—peace of mind.

Forget your previous prejudices against these devices. If you've never tried them before, now is the time. If you've tried them before and didn't like the experience, it is time to try again. The market is now flooded with condoms in all shapes and sizes and colors and flavors. Some are extra tight at the base to restrict leakage after intercourse, and possibly prolong the time to ejaculation. Some are ribbed to enhance pleasure. They are easy to obtain in drug stores, convenience stores, or even by mail order. No prescription is required. They can be used only as needed, thereby avoiding the need for pills or devices that require advance planning and need to be present between episodes of intercourse. Condoms require no premeditation. They can be carried "just in case." Furthermore, the couple committed to making these work for them will find little to diminish the pleasure of making love. They are easy to use and can actually be made a part of the lovemaking process, possibly even enhancing the sexual experience.

Condoms work. They prevent disease and pregnancy. Previously reported failure rates of up to 10 percent are highly inflated. Most of these numbers include people who have used the sheath improperly or who sometimes forgot to use it at all. In fact, in a recent study of physicians using condoms for birth control, no pregnancies were found, once again suggesting that misuse is a more likely cause for failure than the device itself. Properly used, the condom prevents pregnancy a bit better than the intrauterine device and the diaphragm and about the same as the birth control pill. Using the right condom in the right way is the only trick.

Will condoms prevent the transmission of infections?

Will condoms help in the prevention of sexually transmitted diseases, and especially herpes simplex virus infection? **Latex condoms,** properly tested at the manufacturer (go for products from reputable companies), will not allow the passage of infectious agents of any kind, including the virus causing acquired immune deficiency syndrome (AIDS), herpes simplex virus, hepatitis B virus, human papillomavirus (causing genital warts), cytomegalovirus, as well as Chlamydia, gonorrhea, syphilis, etc. The same may not be true for some of the "natural" condoms made from the intestines of animals. These membranes are more variable in their pore sizes, and while perfectly good at preventing pregnancy, they *may* not be as good at preventing disease. Further scientific work needs to be done to sort out the subtle differences between one type and another. For now, in trying to prevent transmission of herpes, go for the ones made from **latex rubber.**

In my opinion, it is preferable to choose a condom containing the **spermicidal agent nonoxynol-9.** This is a safe, soaplike substance that kills sperm. It also kills the herpes virus and the AIDS virus in the test tube, and is, in fact, even being tested as a possible antiviral treatment, in combination with other drugs! Therefore nonoxynol-9 is a second possible prevention tool to be used in combination with the condom. One study showed that even if a condom broke, the AIDS virus (HIV) was inactivated two-thirds of the time by nonoxynol-9 when it was present in the tip of the condom. Nonoxynol-9 can also be used by the woman or recipient partner as a contraceptive foam, serving to aid lubrication and further prevent disease transmission.

Are there any special precautions to take?

Yes. Nothing replaces common sense. Remember these points:

- Condoms cover the penis—the shaft and the tip (glans). They do not cover the base of the shaft, the scrotum, or the pubic hair areas, which are commonly contacted during sexual relations. *It is therefore unwise* to have genital sexual contact during the active phases of infection whether you elect to use a condom or not.
- Furthermore, although using a condom during the *inactive* phases of infection will prevent nearly all herpes transmission, nothing can be called a *guarantee*. In the unlikely event of asymptomatic shedding in vaginal secretions, where the nonoxynol-9 did not inactivate the virus, and where secretions remained at the base of the penis for a prolonged period after intercourse, it is still *possible* to transmit this infection. The statistics here are now getting low enough, however, to make this a rare problem from a practical point of view.
- Condom breakage may occur because of a manufacturing defect. However, tests performed by the major manufacturers make this extremely unlikely. Look for the words "electronically tested" on the package, as a sign of extra concern by the manufacturer. Causes for breakage unrelated to manufacturing problems are much more common and easy to

avoid. These include inadequate lubrication (the most common); use of the wrong lubrication, which weakens the device (see below); use of old and deteriorated condoms or ones that have been left in the heat or sunlight or allowed to dry out because of a previous tear in the package. In addition, condoms may be torn accidentally with teeth, fingernails, or jewelry.

Are there some simple guidelines to follow?

Dr. Robert Hatcher is a professor of gynecology and obstetrics at Emory University School of Medicine. His book, *Contraceptive Technology 1986–1987,* [1] is recommended for further information. He offers "rules" of "condom sense." I have liberally added to and/or edited these for this book, since the transmission of genital herpes is unique among the sexually transmitted infections. Selected advice gleaned from work by Ansell Inc., Dotham, Alabama, and les Départements de santé communautaire du Québec are also incorporated into my version of these rules:

1. If you elect to use condoms for preventing virus transmission, use a quality latex product only. If you are unsure about products, ask the pharmacist or your physician which brands are preferred. Use the condom every single time you have intercourse. *There should be no exceptions.*

2. Put the condom on as soon as erection occurs. *Unprotected contact with any orifice—vagina, mouth, or rectum—is the same as not using a condom at all* from the point of view of transmission. In other words, it is not sufficient to put on the condom after you have begun having intercourse but before ejaculation. If you desire to protect yourself and your partner against all sexually transmitted infections (generally a wise concept), then you would want to avoid unprotected contact altogether, whether this is genital-genital, genital-oral, oral-anal, or whatever. Virtually all

[1]13th ed. (New York: Irvington, 1987)

sexually transmitted infections other than genital herpes are not periodic. If present, transmission could occur during any sexual contact.

3. If your only reason for using condoms is to prevent asymptomatic transmission of genital herpes, then refer also to Chapter 5 on transmission, which discusses these issues in great detail. Since genital herpes is periodic, with active and inactive phases, unprotected contact (e.g., oral-genital) is unlikely to result in transmission during inactive phases of infection. Your choice about unprotected oral-genital contact, and so on, should be based upon a variety of factors mutually discussed with your partner. However, if you and your partner have decided to use condoms to prevent asymptomatic transmission of genital herpes, then mixing protected genital sexual contact with unprotected oral-genital contact is inconsistent.

4. Squeeze any air out of the tip of the condom by holding the tip between the fingers of one hand as you put it on. Air bubbles tend to interfere with sensitivity and may induce breakage.

5. Place the condom on the penis *only after* erection occurs, but *before any* contact between penis and partner. *Then* roll the condom's rim all the way to the base of the penis before insertion into your partner. Do not unroll the condom before putting it on.

6. If the condom lacks a reservoir tip, leave a small empty space (about half an inch) at the tip to catch semen. Better yet, use a condom with a built-in reservoir tip. (Remember to keep the air out of the reservoir tip by squeezing it as you put it on.)

7. For lubrication, do not use petroleum jelly, mineral oil, vegetable shortening or oil, or any other oil-based lubricant, because these may deteriorate the latex. Saliva is also *not* an appropriate lubricant. Sufficient lubrication is essential to prevent the condom from tearing. Most people prefer to purchase prelubricated condoms. If further lubrication is required, use water, or spermicidal jelly or spermicidal foam (preferably containing nonoxynol-9).

Maximum protection calls for using nonoxynol-9, either as part of the condom lubricant, or as a component of the partner's foam, jelly, or cream, or (best choice) as a component of both.

8. After intercourse, hold onto the rim of the condom as the penis is withdrawn, being careful not to spill any of its contents. Withdraw the penis from the partner soon after ejaculation, because as the erection is lost, the condom may slip off, allowing semen to escape.

9. Do not use a condom more than once. A condom is never washable and/or reusable. Dispose of it safely so that no one (a child, for example) has access to it.

10. Store condoms in a cool, dry place. Do not keep them in a wallet, a glove compartment, a dashboard, or other hot place for a long time, because heat can deteriorate the latex. Condoms keep well in a purse or shirt/jacket pocket.

11. Most companies are now putting expiry dates on the condom box. Check for it, and make sure the dates are appropriate.

12. Do not hesitate to open a condom package on your own before using one during a sexual encounter. Check to see what a condom looks like and feels like, and how it unrolls, etc.

13. There is *no evidence,* at this time, that the standard condom will resist breakage during anal sex. New brands composed of a thicker latex are beginning to appear on the market for this purpose, but clinical studies verifying that special brands are required, or, on the other hand, that they work, have yet to be published.

What does the term "safe sex" really mean?

Recently, we have been inundated with material suggesting the practice of "safe sex" to prevent the transmission of all sexually transmitted diseases. The AIDS epidemic, of course, is the main stimulus behind this effort. Such an approach should be supported vigorously in an attempt to control infection. However, the term "safe sex" can be misleading. If a condom is used incorrectly or left in the drawer, barrier contraception provides no benefit. All the techniques of safe sex, definitely enhance—indeed, *markedly* enhance—the safety of sex in general. They make sex *safer*. They do *not* make sex 100 percent safe. Condoms prevent the transmission of most diseases which might otherwise result from penile-vaginal sex. Since this is the most common type of sexual contact, they make most sexual contact a lot safer.

However, a reduction in AIDS or herpes transmission will only come about when safer sexual methods are combined with a reduction in the number of sexual partners. Remember, however, that being selective with a partner does not mean that you should avoid someone who is honest enough to tell you that he or she has genital herpes. Being selective does not mean (from the infectious disease point of view) that you are safe from infection if you feel that you are in love. This is certainly a good start in building a relationship, but other factors should be borne in mind when trying to prevent infection. Sexually transmitted diseases very often cause no obvious symptoms and they do not limit themselves to people who are not lovable. Therefore, if your partner is in a high risk group for sexually transmitted infections other than AIDS (i.e., if their previous sexual partners have been very high in number or occasionally anonymous or casual), then examination for sexually transmitted infection by a competent health care provider is indicated, preferably before having sex, especially before having unprotected sex. If any genital symptoms are present, regardless of how mild, then the same rules should apply. Such examinations are easy to obtain nowadays and should be encouraged. As you already know from reading this book, a clean bill of health on one examination does not rule out genital herpes. However, it can rule out nearly everything else, if done properly. The genital herpes part is dealt with through straightforward rules outlined throughout this book.

If your partner is in a risk group for AIDS, it is easy, anonymous, and usually free of charge to find out if he or she is infected with the AIDS virus. These risk groups include people with the following:

- Any homosexual or bisexual male sexual contact (since 1976).
- Any history of intravenous drug use since 1976.
- A history of receiving unscreened blood products, including transfusions or hemophilia factors since 1976. Most exposure via this route has now ceased to exist because of donor-screening, which began in March/April of 1985.
- A history of sexual contact with a prostitute since 1976.
- A history of sexual contact with a native of one of many Central African countries and/or Haiti.
- A history of being a sexual partner of anyone in a high-risk group listed above.

Find out *before* you have sexual contact. That is safe. Not finding out and having sex with a condom is safer than not using the condom. In fact, the condom method is safer by a factor of 10 times or more, based on transmission studies with AIDS in long-term relationships. Even so, if you seek 100 percent safe sex, you are advised to delay sex until you know whether your partner carries the AIDS virus. Furthermore, one AIDS test alone is only adequate if the reason for the partner's high-risk has ceased to exist. If the partner's exposure is ongoing, the test will *not* provide ongoing reassurance of safety.

If herpes is your only concern regarding transmission, remember that even without condoms, careful attention to the active phases of infection is an effective means of preventing transmission. Using condoms properly during inactive phases offers added protection, making transmission extremely unlikely to occur.

ADDITIONAL SUGGESTED READING

The following list of books and articles on the subject of herpes is recommended for those who wish to read more. This list is not intended to be a complete bibliography or reference section for this book. You will need to visit a medical library for access to all of these articles except those with an asterisk (*). They are selected for inclusion in this section because they are, more or less, readable by a nonprofessional.

To find a medical library, you may call your local medical society and ask. Often the society or local hospital will have their own. A trip to a university with a medical school is occasionally necessary. Call locally first, because often a local small library will be able to obtain a copy of an article on a specific subject by interlibrary loan.

General Topics: Herpes Simplex Virus

Kaplan, A. S., ed. *The Herpes Viruses.* New York: Academic Press, 1973.

Nahmias, A. J.; Dowdle, W. R.; and Schinazi, R. F., eds. *The Human Herpes Viruses: An Interdisciplinary Perspective.* New York: Elsevier North Holland, 1981.

Nahmias, A. J., and Roizman, B. "Infection with Herpes Simplex Viruses 1 and 2." *New England Journal of Medicine* 289 (1973): 667–674, 719–725, 781–789.

Genital Herpes Infection

Adams, H. G., et al. "Genital Herpetic Infection in Men and Women. Clinical Course and Effect of Topical Application of Adenine Arabinoside." *The Journal of Infectious Diseases* 133 Supplement (1976): A151–A159.

Barton, S. E., et al. "Screening to Detect Asymptomatic Shedding of Herpes Simplex Virus (HSV) in Women With Recurrent

Genital HSV Infection." *Genitourinary Medicine* 62 (1986): 181–185.

Bernstein, D. I., et al. "Serologic Analysis of First-Episode Nonprimary Genital Herpes Simplex Virus Infection: Presence of Type 2 Antibody in Acute Serum Samples." *The American Journal of Medicine* 77 (1984): 1055–1060.

Brown, Z. A., et al. "Clinical and Virologic Course of Herpes Simplex Genitalis." *Western Journal of Medicine* 130 (1979): 414–421.

Corey, L. "The Diagnosis and Treatment of Genital Herpes." *Journal of the American Medical Association* 248 (1982): 1041–1049.

Corey, L., et al. "Genital Herpes Simplex Infections: Clinical Manifestations, Course, and Complications." *Annals of Internal Medicine* 98 (1983): 958–972.

Guinan, M. E., et al. "The Course of Untreated Recurrent Genital Herpes Simplex Infection in 27 Women." *New England Journal of Medicine* 304 (1981): 759–763.

Harger, J. H., et al. "Changes in the Frequency of Genital Herpes Recurrences as a Function of Time." *Obstetrics and Gynecology* 67 (1986): 637–642.

Lafferty, W.E., et al. "Recurrences After Oral and Genital Herpes Simplex Virus Infection: Influence of Site Infection and Viral Type." *New England Journal of Medicine* 316 (1987): 1444–1449.

Rooney, J. F., et al. "Acquisition of Genital Herpes from an Asymptomatic Sexual Partner." *New England Journal of Medicine* 314 (1986): 1561–1564.

Sacks, S. L. "Frequency and Duration of Patient-observed Recurrent Genital Herpes Simplex Virus Infection: Characterization of the Nonlesional Prodrome." *Journal of Infectious Dis-*

eases 150 (1984): 873–877.

Sacks, S. L., and Koss, M. "The Emotional and Physical Consequences of Genital Herpes Simplex Virus Infection." *Programs and Abstracts of the 26th Interscience Conference on Antimicrobial Agents and Chemotherapy*. Washington: American Society for Microbiology, 1986.

Sacks, S. L., et al. "Clinical Course of Recurrent Genital Herpes and Treatment with Foscarnet Cream: Results of a Canadian Multicenter Trial." *Journal of Infectious Diseases* 155 (1987): 178–186.

Stenzel-Poore, M.P., et al. "Herpes Simplex Virus Shedding in Genital Secretions." *Sexually Transmitted Diseases* 14 (1987): 17–22.

Vontver, L. A., et al. "Clinical Course and Diagnosis of Genital Herpes Simplex Virus Infection and Evaluation of Topical Surfactant Therapy." *American Journal of Obstetrics and Gynecology* (1979): 548–554.

Herpes of the Newborn

Bradley, J. S., et al. "Neutralization of Herpes Simplex Virus by Antibody in Amniotic Fluid." *Obstetrics and Gynecology* 60 (1982): 318–321.

Brown, Z.A., et al. "Effects on Infants of a First Episode of Genital Herpes During Pregnancy." *New England Journal of Medicine* 317 (1987): 1246–1251.

Committee on Fetus and Newborn. Committee on Infectious Diseases. "Perinatal Herpes Simplex Virus Infections." *Pediatrics* 66 (1980): 147–149.

Harger, J. H., et al. "Characteristics and Management of Pregnancy in Women With Genital Herpes Simplex Virus Infection." *American Journal of Obstetrics and Gynecology* (1983): 784–791.

Honig, P. J., et al. "Congenital Herpes Simplex Virus Infections." *Archives of Dermatology* 115 (1979): 1329–1333.

Kibrick, S. "Herpes Simplex Infection at Term. What To Do With Mother, Newborn and Nursery Personnel." *Journal of the American Medical Association* 243 (1980): 157–160.

Nahmias, A. J.; Keyserling, H. L.; and Kerrick, G. M. "Herpes Simplex." *Infectious Diseases of the Fetus and Newborn Infant.* Edited by J. S. Remington and J. O. Klein. Philadelphia: W. B. Saunders, 1983.

Vontver, L. A., et al. "Recurrent Genital Herpes Simplex Virus Infection in Pregnancy: Infant Outcome and Frequency of Asymptomatic Recurrences." *American Journal of Obstetrics and Gynecology* 143 (1982): 75–81.

Yeager, A. S., et al. "Relationship of Antibody to Outcome in Neonatal Herpes Simplex Virus Infections." *Infection and Immunity* 29 (1980): 532–538.

Herpes and Cancer

Barnett, R., and Fox, R. *A Feminist Approach To Pap Tests.* Available for 50 ¢ postage from the Vancouver Women's Health Collective, 1501 West Broadway, Vancouver, B.C. V6J 1W6.*

Kaufman, R. H., et al. "Herpes Virus-induced Antigens in Squamous Cell Carcinoma In Situ of the Vulva." *New England Journal of Medicine* 305 (1981): 483–488.

Nahmias, A. J., and Sawanabori, S. "The Genital Herpes —Cervical Cancer Hypothesis—10 Years Later." *Progress in Experimental Tumor Research* 21 (1978): 117–139.

Rawls, W. E., et al. "An Analysis of Seroepidemiological Studies of Herpes Virus Type 2 and Carcinoma of the Cervix." *Cancer Research* 33 (1973): 1477–1482.

Schachter, J. "Sexually Transmitted Infections and Cervical Atypia." *Sexually Transmitted Diseases* 8 (1981): 353–356.

Herpes and Psychology

Bok, S. *Lying: Moral Choice in Public and Private Life.* New York: Pantheon Books, 1978.*

Bok, S. *Secrets: On the Ethics of Concealment and Revelation.* New York: Pantheon Books, 1983.*

Kubler-Ross, E. *On Death and Dying.* New York: MacMillan, 1969.*

Selye, H. *Stress Without Distress.* Signet Books: New York, 1975.*

Nongenital Herpes

Bader, C., et al. "The Natural History of Recurrent Facial-Oral Infection with Herpes Simplex Virus." *Journal of Infectious Diseases* 138 (1978): 897–905.

Cavanagh, H. D. "Herpetic Ocular Disease; Therapy of Persistent Epithelial Defects." *International Ophthalmology Clinics* 15 (1975): 67–88.

Gill, M.J., et al. "Herpes Simplex Virus Infection of the Hand: A Profile of 79 Cases." *The American Journal of Medicine* 84 (1988): 89–93.

Wassilew, S. W. "Treatment of Herpes Simplex of the Skin: Critical Evaluation of Antiherpetic Drugs With Reference to Relative Potency On the Eye." *Advances in Ophthalmology* 38 (1979): 125–133.

Whitley, R. J., et al. "Adenine Arabinoside Therapy of Biopsy-proved Herpes Simplex Encephalitis: National Institute of Allergy and Infectious Diseases Collaborative Antiviral Study." *New England Journal of Medicine* 297 (1977): 289–294.

Therapy

Allen, W. P., and Rapp, F. "Concept Review of Genital Herpes Vaccines." *Journal of Infectious Diseases* 145 (March, 1982): 413–421.

Ashley, R. L., and Corey, L. "Effect of Acyclovir Treatment of Primary Genital Herpes on the Antibody Response to Herpes Simplex Virus." *Journal of Clinical Investigations* 73 (1984): 681–688.

Bernstein, D. I.; Lovett, M. A.; and Bryson, Y. J. "The Effects of Acyclovir on Antibody Response to Herpes Simplex Virus in Primary Genital Herpetic Infections." *Journal of Infectious Diseases* 150 (1984): 7–13.

Boyd, M.R., et al. "The Persistent Activity of BRL39123 Against Human Herpes Viruses." *Program and Abstracts of the VIIth International Congress of Virology* (August 1987).

Bryson, Y. J.; Dillon, M.; Lovett, M.; et al. "Treatment of First Episodes of Genital Herpes Simplex Virus Infection With Oral Acyclovir. A Randomized Double-Blind Controlled Trial in Normal Subjects." *New England Journal of Medicine* 16 (1983): 916–921.

Corey, L., and Holmes, K. K. "Genital Herpes Simplex Virus Infections: Current Concepts in Diagnosis, Therapy and Prevention." *Annals of Internal Medicine* 98 (1983): 973–983.

Douglas, J. M.; Critchlow, D.; Benedetti, J.; et al. "A Double-Blind Study of Oral Acyclovir for Suppression of Recurrences of Genital Herpes Simplex Virus Infection." *New England Journal of Medicine* 310 (1984): 1551–1556.

Elion, G. B. "Mechanism of Action and Selectivity of Acyclovir." *American Journal of Medicine* 73 (1982): 7–13.

Elion, G. B.; Furman, P. A.; Fyfe, J. A.; et al. "Selectivity of Action of an Antiherpetic Agent, 9-(2-Hydroxyethoxymethyl)

Guanine." *Proceedings of the National Academy of Science, USA* 74 (1977): 5716–5720.

Furman, P. A.; de Miranda, P.; St. Clair, M. H.; and Elion, G. B. "Metabolism of Acyclovir in Virus-infected and Uninfected Cells." *Antimicrobial Agents and Chemotherapy* 20 (1981): 518–524.

Guinan, M. E. "Therapy for Symptomatic Genital Herpes Simplex Virus Infection: A Review." *Reviews of Infectious Diseases* 4, Supplement (November–December, 1982): 5819–5828.

Luby, J. "Therapy in Genital Herpes." *New England Journal of Medicine,* 306 (June 3, 1982): 1356–1357.

Luby, J., et al. "A Study of Patient-initiated Topical Acyclovir Versus Placebo in the Therapy of Recurrent Genital Herpes." *Journal of Infectious Diseases* 150 (1984): 1–6.

Mertz, G. J., et al. "Double-Blind Placebo Controlled Trial of Oral Acyclovir in First-Episode Genital Herpes Simplex Virus Infection." *Journal of the American Medical Association* 252 (1984): 1147–1151.

Mindel, A.; Faherty, A.; Hindley, A.; et al. "Prophylactic Oral Acyclovir in Recurrent Genital Herpes." *The Lancet* II (1984): 57–59.

Reichman, R. C.; Badger, G. J.; Mertz, G. J.; et al. "Treatment of Recurrent Genital Herpes Simplex Infections with Oral Acyclovir. A Controlled Trial." *Journal of the American Medical Association* 251 (1984): 2103–2117.

Sacks, S. L. "A New Era of Treatment for Herpes Begins with the Licensing of Oral Acyclovir. Make Up Your Own Mind." *The Helper.* Herpes Resource Center, Palo Alto, California (Summer, 1985).

Sacks, S. L. "The Role of Oral Acyclovir in the Management of

Genital Herpes Simplex." *Canadian Medical Association Journal* 136 (1987): 701–707.

Sacks, S. L., et al. "Recombinant Alpha-2 Interferon Gel in the Treatment of Recurrent Herpes Genitalis." *Program and Abstracts of the VIIth International Congress of Virology* (August 1987).

Sacks, S. L., et al. "Six Months Chronic Suppression Compared with Intermittent Lesional Therapy of Frequently Recurring Genital Herpes Using Oral Acyclovir: Effects on Lesions and Nonlesional Prodromes." *Sexually Transmitted Diseases*, in press.

Sacks, S. L., et al. "Suppression of Visible Lesions of Genital Herpes Simplex Recurrences During Chronic Dosing with Oral Acyclovir." *Recent Advances in Chemotherapy.* Edited by J. Ishigami. Tokyo: University of Tokyo Press, 1986.

Sacks, S. L., et al. "Topical 3% Edoxudine Cream in the Treatment of Recurrent Genital Herpes Infection." *Program and Abstracts of the VIIth International Congress of Virology* (August 1987).

Sacks, S. L., et al. "Topical 3% Edoxudine (EDU) for Recurrent Genital and Non-Genital Type 2 Herpes Simplex Virus (HSV) Infection." *Programs and Abstracts of the 27th Interscience Conference on Antimicrobial Agents and Chemotherapy.* Washington: American Society for Microbiology, 1987.

Straus, E. E.; Takiff, H. E.; Seidlin, M.; et al. "Suppression of Frequently Recurring Genital Herpes. A Placebo-controlled Double-Blind Trial of Oral Acyclovir." *New England Journal of Medicine* 310 (1984): 1545–1550.

Wise, T. G., et al. "Herpes Simplex Vaccines." *Journal of Infectious Diseases* 136 (1977): 706–710.

PERMISSIONS

The quotation from *Suzanne Takes You Down* by Leonard Cohen is used by permission of the Canadian Publishers, McClelland and Stewart, Toronto. Lewis Thomas' quotation is from *The Lives Of A Cell* by Lewis Thomas. Copyright © 1974 by Lewis Thomas. All rights reserved. Reprinted by permission of Viking Penguin Inc. The quotation from Richard Selzer is from his book *Mortal Lessons,* copyright © 1974, 1975, 1976 by Richard Selzer. Reprinted by permission of Simon & Schuster, Inc. Alfred A. Knopf, Inc. and Pantheon Books, a Division of Random House, Inc. have courteously granted permission to use quotations from *The Second Sex* by Simone de Beauvoir, translated and edited by H. M. Parshley, copyright © 1974, and from *Secrets: On the Ethics of Concealment and Revelation* by Sissela Bok, copyright © 1982. The following are reprinted by permission of Farrar, Straus and Giroux, Inc. Excerpt from *Cancer Ward* by Aleksandr Solzhenitsyn. English Translation copyright © 1968, 1969 by The Bodley Head Ltd. Excerpt from *Illness as Metaphor* by Susan Sontag. Copyright © 1977, 1978 by Susan Sontag. The quotation from Thomas Szasz comes from his book *Sex by Prescription,* by permission of Doubleday, a division of Bantam, Doubleday, Dell Publishing Group, Inc. Permission to use *Sex and Destiny: The Politics of Human Fertility* by Germaine Greer has been granted by Martin, Secker & Warburg Limited and by Aitken & Stone Limited.

INDEX

Index

Cold sores, 22, 34, 37, 39, 41, 53, 58, 77–79, 81, 85, 92, 93–94, 99, 124, 135–136, 137–139, 145

Colposcopy, 109, 110

Condoms, 17, 76–77, 84, 192–200

Cone biopsy, 110

Congenital herpes, 19; see also Newborn, herpes of the

Conjunctivitis, 90, 141–142

Constipation, 131

Contact lenses, 79, 139

Contagiousness, 17–18, 74–86; see also Active phases of infection; Transmission

Contraceptive foam, 84, 188–189, 197–198; see also Nonoxynol-9

Coping with herpes, 119–122

Crusts, 40, 42, 45, 49, 51, 52

CT scan (Computerized Tomography), 146

Culture test
  in diagnosis, 48, 57, 65–71, 68, 82, 96–97, 148
  historical aspects, 25
  methods, 26
  in pregnancy, 19, 96–97

Cytomegalovirus, 34, 105, 175, 194

Cytopathic effect, 68

Dentists, 135, 139

Diagnosis, clinical, 119, 148; see also Diagnosis, laboratory
  differential, 44
  encephalitis, 146–147
  genital herpes, 65–73
  keratitis, 142–143
  in newborn, 90–91
  syphilis, 57

Diagnosis, laboratory, 22, 25–26, 36, 68, 73; see also Antibody test; Blood test; Culture test; Diagnosis, clinical; DNA fingerprinting; Fluorescent antibody technique; Pap test; Tzanck smear

Discharge, 57, 67, 92, 131

DNA, 27–29, 32, 73, 83, 154–158, 164, 166, 175–176, 180

DNA fingerprinting, 73, 83–84

Drug trials, see Treatments, clinical trials

Drugs, see Treatments, drugs

Dysplasia (of cervix), 110

EB virus, see Epstein-Barr virus

Eczema herpeticum, 134–135, 168

EEG (Electroencephalography), 146

Electron microscopy, 69–70

Emotions
  anger, 57–58, 111, 115–117, 120, 121
  depression, 57–58, 117–118, 121–122
  fear, 57–58, 113, 120, 123, 125–126
  guilt, 53, 112, 115, 119
  shame, 112–114
  shock, 111–112, 120

Encephalitis, 34, 79, 89, 144–147

Envelope, 27–29, 34, 70, 74

Epidural anesthesia, 101

Epstein-Barr virus, 34

Erection, difficulties with, see Impotence

Erythema multiforme, 62–63, 168

Experimental, see Treatments, clinical trials

Eye infections, 39, 76, 77–79, 89, 90, 140–144

Fatal herpes infections, 133

Fetal scalp monitor, 90, 97

Fever, 38, 46, 61, 131, 146

Fever blisters, see Cold sores

Finger infections (Whitlow), 37, 39, 77, 92–93, 135–136, 139, 170

First episode of infections, 37–41, 59, 158–159; see also Primary herpes

Fluorescein dye, 143

Fluorescent antibody technique, 69–70

Foreskin, 38, 43, 44, 48, 104

Frequency of recurrences, 45, 54, 133–134

Ganciclovir, 174–175

Ganglion, 31–32, 35, 41, 55, 58, 76, 133–134, 145, 151, 164

Index

Index

Order Form

If you cannot obtain a copy of this book from a bookstore you may use this order form.

Send To: (please print)

Name _____

Address _____

City _____Province/State _____

Postal/Zip Code _____

Please send me _____ copies of *The Truth About Herpes* by Stephen L. Sacks, M.D.

Total amount enclosed_____

☐ Cheque/money order enclosed, payable to
Gordon Soules Book Publishers Ltd.
☐ Visa   ☐ MasterCard   ☐ American Express
Card No. _____ Expiry Date _____

In the United States, return this form to:

> Gordon Soules Book Publishers Ltd.
> 620 - 1916 Pike Place
> Seattle, WA 98101
>
> price per copy in the U.S.A.: $14.95 — add postage and handling: $2.00 first book, 75¢ for each additional book

In Canada, return this form to:

> Gordon Soules Book Publishers Ltd.
> 1352-B Marine Drive
> West Vancouver, B.C.
> V7T 1B5
>
> price per copy in Canada: $14.95 — add postage and handling: $2.00 first book, 75¢ for each additional book

Order Form

If you cannot obtain a copy of this book from a bookstore you may use this order form.

Send To: (please print)

Name _____

Address _____

City _____Province/State _____

Postal/Zip Code _____

Please send me _____ copies of *The Truth About Herpes* by Stephen L. Sacks, M.D.

Total amount enclosed_____

☐ Cheque/money order enclosed, payable to
Gordon Soules Book Publishers Ltd.
☐ Visa   ☐ MasterCard   ☐ American Express
Card No. _____ Expiry Date _____

In the United States, return this form to:

> Gordon Soules Book Publishers Ltd.
> 620 - 1916 Pike Place
> Seattle, WA 98101
>
> price per copy in the U.S.A.: $14.95 — add postage and handling: $2.00 first book, 75¢ for each additional book

In Canada, return this form to:

> Gordon Soules Book Publishers Ltd.
> 1352-B Marine Drive
> West Vancouver, B.C.
> V7T 1B5
>
> price per copy in Canada: $14.95 — add postage and handling: $2.00 first book, 75¢ for each additional book

Order Form

If you cannot obtain a copy of this book from a bookstore you may use this order form.

Send To: (please print)

Name _____

Address _____

City _____ Province/State _____

Postal/Zip Code _____

Please send me _____ copies of *The Truth About Herpes* by Stephen L. Sacks, M.D.

Total amount enclosed_____

☐ Cheque/money order enclosed, payable to
Gordon Soules Book Publishers Ltd.
☐ Visa ☐ MasterCard ☐ American Express
Card No. _____ Expiry Date _____

In the United States, return this form to:

> Gordon Soules Book Publishers Ltd.
> 620 - 1916 Pike Place
> Seattle, WA 98101
>
> price per copy in the U.S.A.: $14.95 — add postage and handling: $2.00 first book, 75¢ for each additional book

In Canada, return this form to:

> Gordon Soules Book Publishers Ltd.
> 1352-B Marine Drive
> West Vancouver, B.C.
> V7T 1B5
>
> price per copy in Canada: $14.95 — add postage and handling: $2.00 first book, 75¢ for each additional book

Order Form

If you cannot obtain a copy of this book from a bookstore you may use
this order form.

Send To: (please print)

Name _____

Address _____

City _____Province/State _____

Postal/Zip Code _____

Please send me _____ copies of *The Truth About Herpes*
by Stephen L. Sacks, M.D.

Total amount enclosed_____

☐ Cheque/money order enclosed, payable to
Gordon Soules Book Publishers Ltd.
☐ Visa   ☐ MasterCard   ☐ American Express
Card No. _____ Expiry Date _____

In the United States, return this form to:

> Gordon Soules Book Publishers Ltd.
> 620 - 1916 Pike Place
> Seattle, WA 98101
>
> price per copy in the U.S.A.: $14.95 — add postage and
> handling: $2.00 first book, 75¢ for each additional book

In Canada, return this form to:

> Gordon Soules Book Publishers Ltd.
> 1352-B Marine Drive
> West Vancouver, B.C.
> V7T 1B5
>
> price per copy in Canada: $14.95 — add postage and handling:
> $2.00 first book, 75¢ for each additional book

Order Form

If you cannot obtain a copy of this book from a bookstore you may use this order form.

Send To: (please print)

Name _____

Address _____

City _____Province/State _____

Postal/Zip Code _____

Please send me _____ copies of *The Truth About Herpes* by Stephen L. Sacks, M.D.

Total amount enclosed_____

☐ Cheque/money order enclosed, payable to
Gordon Soules Book Publishers Ltd.
☐ Visa   ☐ MasterCard   ☐ American Express
Card No. _____ Expiry Date _____

In the United States, return this form to:

> Gordon Soules Book Publishers Ltd.
> 620 - 1916 Pike Place
> Seattle, WA 98101
>
> price per copy in the U.S.A.: $14.95 — add postage and handling: $2.00 first book, 75¢ for each additional book

In Canada, return this form to:

> Gordon Soules Book Publishers Ltd.
> 1352-B Marine Drive
> West Vancouver, B.C.
> V7T 1B5
>
> price per copy in Canada: $14.95 — add postage and handling: $2.00 first book, 75¢ for each additional book

Order Form

If you cannot obtain a copy of this book from a bookstore you may use this order form.

Send To: (please print)

Name _____

Address _____

City _____Province/State _____

Postal/Zip Code _____

Please send me _____ copies of *The Truth About Herpes* by Stephen L. Sacks, M.D.

Total amount enclosed_____

☐ Cheque/money order enclosed, payable to Gordon Soules Book Publishers Ltd.
☐ Visa   ☐ MasterCard   ☐ American Express
Card No. _____ Expiry Date _____

In the United States, return this form to:

      Gordon Soules Book Publishers Ltd.
      620 - 1916 Pike Place
      Seattle, WA 98101

      price per copy in the U.S.A.: $14.95 — add postage and handling: $2.00 first book, 75¢ for each additional book

In Canada, return this form to:

      Gordon Soules Book Publishers Ltd.
      1352-B Marine Drive
      West Vancouver, B.C.
      V7T 1B5

      price per copy in Canada: $14.95 — add postage and handling: $2.00 first book, 75¢ for each additional book

Order Form

If you cannot obtain a copy of this book from a bookstore you may use this order form.

Send To: (please print)

Name _____

Address _____

City _____Province/State _____

Postal/Zip Code _____

Please send me _____ copies of *The Truth About Herpes* by Stephen L. Sacks, M.D.

Total amount enclosed_____

☐ Cheque/money order enclosed, payable to
Gordon Soules Book Publishers Ltd.
☐ Visa   ☐ MasterCard   ☐ American Express
Card No. _____ Expiry Date _____

In the United States, return this form to:

>   Gordon Soules Book Publishers Ltd.
>   620 - 1916 Pike Place
>   Seattle, WA 98101
>
>   price per copy in the U.S.A.: $14.95 — add postage and handling: $2.00 first book, 75¢ for each additional book

In Canada, return this form to:

>   Gordon Soules Book Publishers Ltd.
>   1352-B Marine Drive
>   West Vancouver, B.C.
>   V7T 1B5
>
>   price per copy in Canada: $14.95 — add postage and handling: $2.00 first book, 75¢ for each additional book

Order Form

If you cannot obtain a copy of this book from a bookstore you may use this order form.

Send To: (please print)

Name _____

Address _____

City _____Province/State _____

Postal/Zip Code _____

Please send me _____ copies of *The Truth About Herpes* by Stephen L. Sacks, M.D.

Total amount enclosed_____

☐ Cheque/money order enclosed, payable to
Gordon Soules Book Publishers Ltd.
☐ Visa   ☐ MasterCard   ☐ American Express
Card No. _____ Expiry Date _____

In the United States, return this form to:

  Gordon Soules Book Publishers Ltd.
  620 - 1916 Pike Place
  Seattle, WA 98101

  price per copy in the U.S.A.: $14.95 — add postage and handling: $2.00 first book, 75¢ for each additional book

In Canada, return this form to:

  Gordon Soules Book Publishers Ltd.
  1352-B Marine Drive
  West Vancouver, B.C.
  V7T 1B5

  price per copy in Canada: $14.95 — add postage and handling: $2.00 first book, 75¢ for each additional book